Guide to the preparation, use and quality assurance of blood components

Recommendation No. R (95) 15

Third edition

Council of Europe Publishing

French edition:

Guide pour la préparation, l'utilisation et l'assurance de qualité des composants sanguins

ISBN 92-871-3195-3

Cover design: Atelier de création graphique, Council of Europe

Council of Europe Publishing
F-67075 Strasbourg Cedex

ISBN 92-871-3196-1
© Council of Europe, 1997
Printed in Germany

CONTENTS

COUNCIL OF EUROPE

COMMITTEE OF MINISTERS

RECOMMENDATION No. R (95) 15

OF THE COMMITTEE OF MINISTERS TO MEMBER STATES

**ON THE PREPARATION, USE AND QUALITY ASSURANCE
OF BLOOD COMPONENTS**

*(Adopted by the Committee of Ministers on 12 October 1995
at the 545th meeting of the Ministers' Deputies)*

The Committee of Ministers, under the terms of Article 15.*b* of the Statute of the Council of Europe;

Considering that the aim of the Council of Europe is to achieve greater unity between its members and that this aim may be pursued, *inter alia*, by the adoption of common action in the health field;

Recalling its Resolution (78) 29 on harmonisation of legislations of member states relating to removal, grafting and transplantation of human substances;

Recalling also its Recommendations No. R (80) 5 concerning blood products for the treatment of haemophiliacs, No. R (81) 14 on preventing the transmission of infectious diseases in the international transfer of blood, its components and derivatives, No. R (84) 6 on the prevention of the transmission of malaria by blood transfusion, No. R (85) 12 on the screening of blood donors for the presence of AIDS markers, No. R (86) 6 on guidelines for the preparation, quality control and use of fresh frozen plasma, No. R (88) 4 on the responsibilities of health authorities in the field of blood transfusion and No. R (93) 4 concerning clinical trials involving the use of components and fractionated products derived from human blood or plasma;

Taking into account the Council Directive 89/381/EEC extending the scope of Directives 65/65/EEC and 75/319/EEC on the approximation of provisions laid down by law, regulation or administrative action relating to proprietary medicinal products and laying down special provisions for medicinal products derived from human blood or human plasma;

Taking into account Agreement No. 26 on the exchange of therapeutic substances of human origin;

Considering the importance of blood components in modern haemotherapy and the necessity to ensure their safety, efficacy and quality;

Considering that such components are of human origin and that hence specific ethical and technical principles have to be taken into account;

Considering the need for harmonisation of such principles in member states;

Considering that biotechnology does not provide substitutes for most blood products;

Convinced, therefore, of the need to provide health authorities, transfusion services as well as hospital blood banks and clinical users with a set of guidelines for the preparation, use and quality assurance of blood components;

Aware that the *Guide to the preparation, use and quality assurance of blood components* published by the Council of Europe has already become the generally-accepted European standard and that it is therefore appropriate to give a legal basis to this guide;

Considering that this guide will be regularly updated by the committee of experts of the Council of Europe,

Recommends that the governments of member states take all necessary measures and steps to ensure that the preparation, use and quality control of blood components are carried out in accordance with the guidelines set out in the appendix[1] to this recommendation.

---

1. The appendix is available from the Publishing and Documentation Service under the reference *Guide to the preparation, use and quality assurance of blood components*, ISBN 92-871-2687-9.

APPENDIX

to the Recommendation No. R (95) 15
on the preparation,
use and quality assurance
of blood components

Introduction

The purpose of this Recommendation is to provide transfusion services with a set of guidelines and principles relating to the preparation, use and quality assurance of blood components.

The requirements set out in this Recommendation are the minimum criteria for the selection of donors. For example, donors with dura mater transplants may be barred from donation subject to National Health Authorities' regulations.

These guidelines and descriptions of the different blood components should also be of value to hospital blood banks and the clinical users of these therapeutic products. As these guidelines were originally and primarily designed to provide information on quality assurance, some relative emphasis is to be expected on this aspect including the selection of donors, the control of laboratory reagents and proficiency testing of staff carrying out the procedures necessary for the safe preparation, selection and transfusion of blood and its components.

This Recommendation covers all of the normal components of blood which will be prepared at a routine blood transfusion service. It does not cover plasma products obtained by fractionation. This aspect of blood transfusion work is the responsibility of the European Pharmacopoeia under the aegis of the Council of Europe and the Commission of the European Communities.

It is inevitable, even in the best of laboratories, that some materials will fail some of the tests, and a strict protocol should be drawn up showing action to be taken in such an eventuality. It is essential that all staff in a blood transfusion service be trained to accept quality control as a welcome and necessary part of everyday work. It is useful to cultivate a positive attitude towards the detection and correction of errors though the emphasis is on the prevention of problems and the production of blood components. A sensible scheme of rotation of junior staff between routine departments and the quality control department may help to foster such an attitude.

Part A:
Good Manufacturing Practice
for blood components

Good Manufacturing Practice for blood components

Because of their intended use, good quality is crucial to blood components. Therefore, the collection of blood and the processing, storage and distribution of blood components must be organised in a way to ensure a high component quality. This can only be achieved if the blood transfusion service has a system of quality management.

Quality management

Quality management is an integrated system of quality assurance covering all matters which individually or collectively influence the components in order to guarantee their quality. Such a system includes *Good Manufacturing Practice* (GMP), *quality control* and an *audit programme,* all of which are closely linked.

GMP encompasses both the processing and quality control of blood components, whereas *internal quality control* and *proficiency testing* are aspects of the quality system concerned with the examination of materials, components, and the proficiency of the staff, in order to ascertain whether they satisfy the defined standards.

The quality requirements involve the following topics:

- quality control and proficiency testing;

- internal and external audits;

- personnel and organisation;

- premises, equipment and materials;

- documentation;

- blood processing;

- complaints and component recall;

- management of errors and accidents.

Quality control and proficiency testing

Generally speaking, quality control refers to activities including steps of verification and testing which are used to assure that materials and processes meet their intended specifications. Proficiency testing is an aspect of Quality Assurance which monitors the ability to perform laboratory procedures within acceptable limits of accuracy through the analysis of unknown specimens distributed by an external source.

The line between quality control and proficiency testing is, in some cases, ill defined. To a great extent, the performance of quality control procedures on components and reagents will be in itself a measure of the proficiency of the staff preparing these components. However, it is accepted that certain procedures are themselves more subject to operative variability, and the institution of proficiency testing exercises in these particular instances is recognised as being necessary. This is particularly the case when the test concerned involves one or more unknowns, as in the case of grouping and cross-matching of blood for hospital patients.

In addition to internal quality control a full programme should also include *external quality control* which should be the task of designated approved laboratories.

Internal and external audits

Internal audits are required to ensure that all procedures and the associated quality control are performed according to the principles of GMP, and should be carried out according to an established programme by persons with well defined responsibilities and authority. *External audits* should also be performed by a designated approved authority.

Personnel and organisation

The preparation of blood components of good quality relies to a great extent upon the individuals doing the work. For this reason, there must be an adequate number of suitably qualified personnel. The tasks and responsibilities of all individuals must be clearly understood and documented. All personnel should be trained in the principles of GMP relevant to their work.

There should be an organisation chart showing the hierarchical structure of the blood transfusion service showing clear delineation of lines of responsibility.

Key personnel in the blood transfusion service includes at least a Production Manager, a Quality Assurance Manager and a Medical Specialist. An individual may have more than one function but the Production Manager and Quality Assurance Manager must be independent of each other.

Personnel should receive initial and continued training appropriate to the duties assigned to them. Training programmes should be available for this purpose. Training records should be kept and the effectiveness of the programmes should be assessed by regular and routine competency evaluation.

Personnel should have relevant knowledge of microbiology, hygiene and GMP and should constantly be aware that microbial contamination of themselves, the donors, the blood components and the environment must be prevented.

Hygiene instructions must be present in each department of the blood transfusion service. These instructions should be understood and strictly followed by all personnel.

Premises, equipment and materials

Premises

Premises must be located, designed, constructed and adapted to suit the operations to be carried out. Their design and furnishing must be chosen to minimise the risk of errors. Premises should, if possible, be designed so that operations can proceed in an orderly manner and crossing lines be avoided. The construction of premises and equipment must permit effective cleaning and maintenance.

The premises should include separate areas for:

-    donor selection;

-    blood collection;

-    blood processing;

-    storage (materials, intermediate and finished blood components);

-    laboratory facilities;

-    auxiliary facilities

Premises to which *donors* have access should be separate from other working areas. There should be separate areas for the selection of donors and the drawing of blood.

Premises for the *preparation of blood components* should be separate from other areas and used exclusively for this purpose. Entry to these areas should be restricted to authorised personnel. Areas for *irradiating* blood components should meet statutory requirements.

Storage areas should be of sufficient capacity to allow orderly storage of the various categories of materials and components. There should be areas for storage of released blood components, separate from other storage areas to prevent any mix-up.

There should be areas for *laboratory testing* and for *quality control.* These areas should be separate from the component preparation areas.

Staff rooms and *canteens* should be separate from other areas. Facilities for *changing clothes* and for *washing* and *toilet* purposes should be adequate.

Equipment

Manufacturing equipment should be designed and maintained to suit its intended purpose and should not present any hazard to donors, components or operators. Periodic maintenance and calibration should be carried out according to established procedures.

Materials

Detailed specifications for purchase of reagents and other materials are required. Only materials that meet the documented requirements should be used. Manufacturers should provide a certificate of compliance for materials such as blood bags, filters, test reagents for infectious disease testing. Equipment and material should conform to international standards where these exist. Inventory records should be kept for traceability and to avoid use after expiry date.

Documentation

Adequate written documentation prevents errors that may result from oral communication. Documentation must enable all manufacturing steps and all data affecting the quality of the components to be checked, from the donor to the recipient of the blood component and vice-versa.

Donors documentation in general and donor deferral records in particular must be subject to the same controls as for documentation of components preparation.

Data can also be stored in 'non-written' form, for instance on computer or microfilm. Users should only have access to those categories of data for which they are authorised.

Documentation should cover at least the following items:

-   a documentation manual;

-   specifications (materials, labels, equipment, blood components, reagents);

-   standard operating procedures (SOPs);

-   other procedures (e.g. manuals, cleaning) ;

-   records on performance of operations (eg notes on donor selection, quality control etc);

-   description of computer hardware and software;

-   protocols (eg audits, complaints);

-   training records on personnel;

-   batch protocols for infrequently used components and materials.

Documents should be approved, dated and signed by appropriate and authorised persons. Documents should not be hand-written except for those parts where data have to be entered. Any alterations made on a hand-written record should be dated and signed.

Documents relating to the selection of donors and the preparation and quality control of blood components should be retained for at least five years or according to local regulations.

If demanded, a document known as Manufacturing Formula and Processing Instructions (MFPI) for each kind of blood component to be manufactured should be prepared. A processing record based on the MFPI should also be kept and this document should be dated and signed by the personnel responsible for component preparation and quality control.

Whenever applicable, records of equipment validation, calibration, maintenance and repairs (and subsequent revalidation) should be maintained.

Blood processing

Donor selection

The final quality of blood components depends on many factors and starts with the selection of donors and blood collection. Donors should be carefully selected according to national regulations. (see also chapters 1 and 2).

Blood collection

The collection procedure should be carefully controlled. The blood bag system must be inspected before use for damage and contamination. Defects of the bag that may adversely affect the quality of the contents must be noted and reported to the quality control department who will be responsible for further action.

Component preparation

Blood components must be prepared in accordance with clear and detailed instructions, and precise adherence to these instructions is required to obtain components of the desired quality. The biological nature of the starting material results in a great degree of variability in the composition of the components. Regular quality control during the processing is therefore of great importance.

Blood components should be processed within a closed system where possible. If a sterile connection device is used, the connection can be regarded as part of the closed system. Processing involving an open system should be carried out in a special area because of risk of microbial contamination.

New processing procedures must be validated before they are introduced and whenever they are altered.

During the whole process all containers of blood or blood components should be clearly labelled. There should be instructions concerning the type of labels and the method of labelling. (see also chapter 3).

Storage, issue and transportation

Final components that have not yet been released for distribution must be kept in quarantine and should be released only when all the required quality controls and laboratory tests have been completed and laboratory results meet the established requirements. Further details for every component are specified in chapter 3.

Contract testing

If certain tasks, such as infectious disease testing, are performed externally, these should be subject to a highly specific written contract. The contract should ensure that the contractor meets GMP requirements.

Complaints and component recall

All complaints and other information that may suggest that defective blood components have been issued must be carefully investigated. Written procedures must exist for recalling defective blood components or blood components suspected of being defective. These written procedures must encompass any look back procedures which may be necessary. All complaints about delivered blood components should be dealt with and investigated as quickly as possible.

The consequences of instituting a full quality control programme should also be borne in mind. Under no circumstances should the quality control laboratory come to be regarded with suspicion by the other workers in the service, and the work of the quality control staff should not be allowed to be viewed by others as being counter-productive to the overall success of the service. It is of course possible that the other, equally counter-productive, extreme may come about whereby complacency is bred in the minds of the routine staff by the assurance that any errors they commit will be picked up further down the line by the quality control staff. A sensible scheme of rotation of junior staff between routine departments and the quality control department may help to overcome these particular difficulties.

Part B: Blood collection

Chapter 1: Selection of donors

Principles of self-sufficiency from voluntary and non-remunerated donations have been recommended and promoted by the Council of Europe and adopted by the European Commission in Directive 39/381 which states (article 3 paragraph 4) that

> "Member States shall take the necessary measures to promote Community *self-sufficiency* in human blood or human plasma. For this purpose, they shall encourage the voluntary unpaid donations of blood and plasma and shall take the necessary measures to develop the production and use of products derived from human blood or plasma coming from voluntary unpaid donations. They shall notify the Commission of such measures."

Donation is considered voluntary and non-remunerated if the person gives blood, plasma or cellular components of his own free will and receives no payment for it, either in the form of cash, or in kind which could be considered a substitute for money. This would include time off work other than that reasonably needed for the donation and travel. Small tokens, refreshments and reimbursements of direct travel costs are compatible with voluntary, non-remunerated donation.

NB: Specific immunisation programmes are not considered in this document but donors enrolled for this purpose should at least fulfil the minimum criteria outlined above (see also *Annex 2, Requirements for the collection, processing and quality control of blood, blood components and plasma derivatives,WHO Technical Report Series, No. 840, 1994.*).

A.   Whole blood donors

In selecting individuals for blood donation the main purpose is to determine whether the person is in good health, in order to protect the donor against damage to his/her own health, and to protect the recipient against transmission of diseases or drugs which could be detrimental to the patient.

Only persons in normal health with a good medical history should be accepted as donors of blood for therapeutic use.

The donor's medical history shall be evaluated, and the donor accepted, by a suitably qualified person trained to use accepted guidelines for selection of blood donors. This person should work under the supervision of a physician. Abnormal conditions should preferably be referred to the physician in charge who should have the final decision on whether blood shall be collected from a donor. If the physician is in doubt the donor should be deferred.

A complete medical and physical examination of blood donors is generally not possible in practice. One has to rely upon the donor's answers to some simple questions concerning his/her medical history and general health, combined with a simple inspection of the donor's appearance and simple laboratory examinations.

To obtain relevant information about the donor's medical history and general health, it is recommended that a preprinted questionnaire be completed.

A locally produced questionnaire should take account of the points listed in the addendum of this chapter.

The questionnaire should be given to all donors.

The questionnaire should be signed by all donors thus certifying that the relevant questions have been asked.

1.   Quantity

A standard donation is 450 mL ± 10%; an optimum blood/anticoagulant ratio is 7 to 1.

2.   Weight

No more than 13% of the estimated blood volume should be taken as whole blood during one blood donation. The blood volume may be estimated from height and weight of the donor. A standard donation should not be collected from persons weighing less than 50 kg.

3.   Interval between donations

It is acknowledged that current practices in some transfusion services in Europe allow up to five standard donations per year to be taken from males and up to four per year from females, with a minimum interval between standard donations of two months.

It is recommended that these donation rates never be exceeded under any circumstances, and be accepted by any transfusion service only after careful consideration of the dietary habits of the populations concerned, and in the knowledge that extra care may be necessary, beyond routine haemoglobin or haematocrit [or Erythrocyte volume fraction (EVF)] estimation, in the monitoring of donors for iron deficiency. It is further recommended that an active donor panel be maintained of sufficient size to allow donors to be bled less often than the maximum rates stated, thus affording the donors extra protection and giving the system flexibility to deal with large-scale emergency situations.

4.   *Age*

Minimum: 18 years.

-    If this is below the legal minimum age of consent, written parental approval will be needed.

Maximum: 65 years.

-    Bleeding donors outside these age limits is at the discretion of the responsible physician, as is the recruitment of any first-time donor above the age of 60.

5.   *Inspection of donor's appearance*

Special note should be taken of plethora, poor physique, debilitation, under-nutrition, anaemia, jaundice, cyanosis, dyspnoea, mental instability, intoxication from alcohol or narcotic drugs.

6.   *Pulse and blood pressure*

It is recommended that pulse and blood pressure be tested routinely. The pulse should be regular and between 50 and 100 beats per minute. It is recognised that recording the blood pressure may be subject to several variables but as a guide the systolic blood pressure should not exceed 180 mm of mercury and the diastolic pressure 100 mm.

7.   *Laboratory examinations*

-    Haemoglobin: should be determined each time the donor presents him/herself, unless substituted by estimation of EVF

- Minimum values before donation:

  Female donors: 125 g per litre 7.4 mmole/litre (min. EVF = 0.38)

  Male donors: 135 g per litre 8.4 mmole/litre (min. EVF = 0.4)

- Donations may be accepted below these levels at the discretion of responsible physicians

- Abnormally high and low values should be further investigated, as should a fall in haemoglobin concentration of more than 20 g/litre between two successive donations.

8.   *Hazardous occupations*

Hazardous occupations or hobbies should normally entail an interval of not less than 12 hours between donation and returning to the occupation or hobby. As examples, such hazardous occupations or hobbies include piloting, bus or train driving, crane operating, climbing of ladders or scaffolding, gliding, climbing and diving.

9.   *Medical history*

- Acquired Immune Deficiency Syndrome (AIDS)

  All blood donors should be provided with accurate and updated information on HIV transmission and AIDS so that those indulging in unsafe sex practices or other risk behaviour exposing them to potential infectious sources will refrain from donating. Blood and blood products with a known confirmed positive marker for HIV should not be used for therapeutic purposes. All blood donors found to have a repeat reactive marker for HIV should be informed, as part of a full counselling procedure, that they should not give further donations.

- Allergy

  Prospective donors with pollen allergy should be deferred during the season: those receiving desensitisation injections should be deferred until 72 hours after the last injection. Donors with local eczema at the venepuncture site should be deferred temporarily. Individuals suffering from asthma which is mild and asymptomatic at the time of donation and requiring only sporadic use of inhalers may be accepted.

- <u>Autoimmune diseases</u>

Causes for rejection, if more than one organ is affected.

- <u>Beta-thalassemia</u>

Heterozygote carriers of beta-thalassemia trait may give blood provided they are in good health and have a haemoglobin level within acceptable values.

- <u>Bronchitis</u>

Persons with symptoms of severe chronic bronchitis should not be accepted as donors.

- <u>Cancer</u>

See malignant diseases.

- <u>Common cold</u>

See infectious diseases.

- <u>Creutzfeldt-Jakob Disease</u>

All individuals who have in the past been treated with extracts derived from human pituitary glands or who have a family history of Creutzfeldt-Jakob Disease are debarred from donation.

Comment:

It is easy to ask donors if they have any family history of CJD: if they say "I do not know what Creutzfeldt-Jakob disease is, you can be practically certain the disease has not occurred in their family, as if it had they would know the name of the disease.

- Diabetes

Permanent rejection if on insulin therapy.

- Drugs

See intoxication.

- Epilepsy

Normally permanent rejection, whether treated or not.

- Fever above 38 °C, flu-like illness

Deferral of at least two weeks following cessation of symptoms.

- Heart and blood vessel disease

Persons with a history of heart disease, especially coronary disease, angina pectoris, severe cardiac arrhythmia, a history of cerebrovascular diseases, arterial thrombosis or recurrent venous thrombosis are excluded. (See also hypertension).

- Hypertension

Hypertensive person whether under treatment or not should not be accepted as a blood donor. The same is true for persons who are being treated with hypotensive drugs and have normal blood pressure (see also 6 *supra*).

- Immunisations

Inoculations, vaccinations: Quarantine period

1.   Vaccines with attenuated bacteria and viruses

BCG, smallpox, yellow fever, rubella
measles, poliomyelitis (oral)   Four weeks

2.   Vaccines with killed bacteria

      Cholera, typhoid (TAB) T   48 hours if well

3.   Vaccines with inactivated viruses

      Poliomyelitis (injection), influenza   48 hours if well

4.   Toxoids

      Diphtheria, tetanus   48 hours if well

5.   Other vaccines

      Hepatitis A vaccine   48 hours if well and no
      Hepatitis B vaccine   exposure (see section on jaundice and
      hepatitis)

      Rabies   48 hours if well
                                               One year if post-exposure

6.   Sera of animal origin   3 months

-     Infectious diseases

      Generally a quarantine of at least two weeks following cessation of symptoms; one
      week in the case of a common cold:

            .   Babesiosis: permanent rejection.

            .   Confirmed brucellosis – rejection for at least two years following full
                  recovery.

.   Leishmaniasis (Kala-Azar): permanent rejection.

.   Toxoplasmosis: quarantine for two years following clinical recovery, provided there is no IgM antibody.

.   Tuberculosis: may be accepted two years after having been declared cured.

.   Contact with an infectious disease: quarantine period = incubation period, or if unknown, nature of contact and period of deferral to be determined by the responsible physician.

-       Intoxication, alcohol and drugs

Persons clearly under the influence of alcohol should be deferred until sober. Illicit drug taking if admitted or suspected (in particular, i.v. drug abuse at any time) must debar.

-       Jaundice and hepatitis

Donors should be provided with up-to-date information on the risk activities which may be associated with hepatitis transmission to provide the opportunity for self-exclusion. Individuals with a history of jaundice or hepatitis may, at the discretion of the appropriate competent medical authority, be accepted as blood donors provided an approved test for HBsAg and anti HCV is negative. Persons whose blood gives a positive reaction for the presence of HBsAg and/or anti-HCV are excluded. Presence of anti-HBs does not debar. Persons who have been in house contact with a case of hepatitis or who have received a transfusion of blood or blood products should have a quarantine period of twelve months. The same is true for acupuncture (other than under strict medical supervision) tattooing and body-piercing. Hospital staff coming into direct contact with patients with hepatitis are accepted at the discretion of the physician in charge of the blood collecting unit providing they have not suffered an inoculation injury involving an infected patient. Donors without demonstrable markers of hepatitis who have donated blood to two patients strongly suspected of having transfusion-transmitted hepatitis should be excluded. The only donor of blood to a recipient with transfusion-transmitted hepatitis should also be excluded.

-       Kidney disease

Acute glomerulonephritis: five years' quarantine period following complete recovery. Chronic nephritis and pyelonephritis: rejection.

- Malignant diseases

Individuals with a malignant disease, or a history of such, are usually permanently excluded. The physician in charge may make exceptions to this rule in selected cases. For example, donors may be accepted at the conclusion of successful treatment for non-invasive cervical cancer and rodent ulcer.

- Medication

Taking of a medication might indicate an underlying disease which may disqualify the donor. It is recommended that a list of commonly used drugs, with rules for acceptability of donors, approved by the medical staff of the transfusion centre, be available to the donor personnel. Donors treated with prescribed drugs should be deferred for a period consistent with the pharmacokinetic properties of the drug.

- Osteomyelitis

Two years after having been declared cured.

- Polycythaemia rubra vera

Rejection.

- Pregnancy

Pregnant women should not be accepted, other than in exceptional circumstances and at the discretion of the physician in charge of the pregnancy. Following pregnancy, the quarantine period should last as many months as the duration of the pregnancy, or at least throughout the lactation period.

- Rheumatic fever

An individual with a history of rheumatic fever should be deferred for two years and then examined for chronic heart sequelae. The latter complication is a cause for rejection.

- <u>Surgery</u>

    Major surgery: generally a quarantine period of six months. Minor surgery (tooth extraction, etc.): one week, if no complications. Persons with a history of resection of the stomach are usually permanently excluded.

- <u>Transfusion</u>

    Donors transfused with blood or blood products should be deferred for twelve months.

- <u>Tropical diseases</u>

    <u>Malaria</u>

i.   Individuals who have lived in a malarial area within the first five years of life are more likely to have sufficient immunity to make them symptomless carriers of the malarial parasite. They may be accepted as blood donors if six months have elapsed since their last visit to an endemic malarious area provided the results of an approved immunologic test for malarial antibodies are negative. If the results are positive, the donor should be permanently rejected as a cellular donor. If an approved antibody test is not available, the individual may be accepted as a blood donor if a symptom-free period of a minimum of three years has elapsed since return from the last visit to an endemic area.

ii. All other persons who have visited an area where malaria is endemic can be accepted as blood donors six months after returning, if they have had no febrile episodes during or after their stay in the malarious area. Individuals having had such febrile episodes can be accepted if the result of an approved immunological test is negative six months after becoming asymptomatic and cessation of therapy. If an approved antibody test is not available, the individual may be accepted as a blood donor if a minimum of a symptom-free period of three years has elapsed since return from the endemic area.

iii. Individuals with a history of diagnosed malaria should be deferred until asymptomatic and off treatment. They may then donate plasma only for three years, and then donate red cells only if an approved antibody test is negative.

iv. The quarantine periods and immunological tests mentioned above may be omitted for those donors whose red cells are discarded and whose plasma is used exclusively for fractionation into blood products, thus rendering it safe from the transmission of malaria. It should be remembered that liquid or frozen untreated plasma and frozen cryoprecipitates cannot be regarded as wholly devoid of the cellular elements of blood and, therefore, of viable malarial parasites.

v. Since questioning of the donor as to the country(ies) in which he was born, brought up or has visited is essential for effective detection, every transfusion service should have a map of the endemic zones and an alphabetical list of the countries concerned.

- Chagas disease

The blood of persons who have resided in areas where the disease is endemic because of unfavourable living conditions should be used only for plasma fractionation products.

- Persons coming or returning from tropical areas should not be accepted as donors until six months after return,and then only if they have not suffered an unexplained fever or illness.

- Unexplained weight loss should be investigated before donation.

B. Apheresis donors

The supervision and medical care of apheresis donors should be the responsibility of a physician specially trained in these techniques.

Other than in exceptional circumstances (to be decided by the responsible physician), donors for apheresis procedures shall meet the usual criteria for ordinary whole blood donations.

In addition, the following criteria should be observed:

1. Medical history

Special attention should be given to the following conditions:

- abnormal bleeding episodes;

- a history suggestive of fluid retention (of special interest if steroids and/or plasma expanders are to be used);

33

-   the taking of drugs containing acetylsalicylic acid within five days prior to thrombocytapheresis;

-   a history of gastric symptoms (if steroids are to be used);

-   adverse reactions to previous donations.

Presence of sickle cell trait will debar.

2.   *Examination of the donor*

i.   Plasmapheresis:

-   evaluation by a physician;

-   pulse, blood pressure, temperature (if required);

-   haemoglobin or haematocrit:

-   protein analysis, such as determination of total serum protein and/or electrophoresis and/or quantitation of single proteins, especially albumin and IgG; total proteins should not be less than 60 g per litre. This analysis should be carried out at suitable intervals but at least annually.

ii.   Additionally on donors undergoing serial plasmapheresis – at suitable intervals but at least annually:

-   evaluation by a physician of the total serum protein values and/or electrophoresis and/or quantitation of single proteins, especially albumin and IgG.

-   Special attention should be paid to any significant fall in these values even though they may still come within the accepted normal limits.

iii.   Cytapheresis:

-   evaluation by a physician;

-       pulse, blood pressure;

-       haemoglobin or haematocrit;

-       for thrombocytapheresis: platelet count – routine thrombocytapheresis should not be carried out on individuals whose normal count is less than 150×10^9 per litre:

3.   *Frequency of donation and maximal amounts of removal of plasma*

-    Not more than 15 litres of plasma should be removed from one donor per year.

-    Not more than 1 litre of plasma should be removed from one donor per week.

-    In the absence of volume replacement not more than 650 mL of plasma should be removed from one donor per apheresis procedure. A suitable form of fluid replacement should be provided if the plasma volume withdrawn in one session exceeds the standard 600-650 mL.

-    Erythrocyte loss should preferably be kept below 20 mL of packed red cells per week.

-    The interval between one apheresis procedure and a whole blood donation should be at least 48 hours. The interval between whole blood donation or failed return of red cells during apheresis, and the next apheresis procedure, should be at least one month.

C.   **Donors of haematopoietic progenitor cells derived from bone marrow or peripheral blood**

1.   *Medical history*

Donors of haematopoietic cells shall meet the health criteria established for normal whole blood donors.

Autologous donors should be similarly evaluated.

In exceptional, life saving situations, some deviation from the normal standards may be necessary, but in these situations the donor, the potential recipient, and their respective physicians should be informed and give their consent.

2.   *Evaluation of the donor*

The prospective donor shall be evaluated for the risks of the collection procedure by a licensed physician other than the physician in charge of the patient (for allogenic donors).

Donors shall be informed about the collective procedures and its potential risks. No serious sequelae have so far been reported following the use of GCSF in normal volunteer donor of peripheral blood progenitor cells, but there is insufficient data available to allow a recommendation on its use to be made.

An informed consent in writing shall be obtained from the donor.

Autologous or peripheral blood cell donors must be tested for transmissible infectious diseases not more than 30 days prior to each donation.

D.   Cord blood donors

A family medical history with particular reference to inherited disease will be obtained.

The prospective maternal donor shall be tested for transmissible infectious diseases not more than 30 days prior to donation. The procedure must be fully explained to the mother who must be put under no pressure to agree to the donation. An informed consent in writing shall be obtained from the prospective maternal donor. The mother must be informed that the cord blood will be used in future potential recipients and will not be reserved for the donor or the donor's family. The pregnancy must be normal throughout and the infant as it is delivered should be checked to ensure that it appears healthy, prior to collection of cord blood. These tests shall be repeated between 6 and 12 months following donation of the cord cells. The infant shall be examined between 6 and 12 months of age for evidence of genetic diseases before the cells may be used for transplantation.

ADDENDUM: FRAMEWORK FOR QUESTIONNAIRE

A questionnaire should be given to all donors each time they come and should be signed by the donor and/or the person who carries out the medical examination.

The questionnaire should contain the following items:

1.   Are you in good health? Have you experienced any of the following:
-    unexpected weight loss
-    unexplained fever
-    swollen glands
-    current medication and recent vaccination, dental treatment

2.   Have you read and understood the information on AIDS and hepatitis?

Do you consider yourself by virtue of your medical history or behaviour and\or health status as a potential risk candidate for the recipient?

3.   Since your last donation, within the previous 12 months have you had:
-    an operation or medical investigation
-    body piercing, tattoo and/or acupuncture other than under medical supervision
-    have you been transfused and/or pregnant?

4.   Have you ever had
-    family history of Creuztfeldt-Jakob Disease (CJD)
-    human pituitary treatment,
-    medication with Accutaine, Tigason, Finasteride

5.   Were you born or have you lived and/or travelled abroad?
-    where?

6.   Have you been exposed to hepatitis?
-    (family or job)

7.   Have you ever suffered from?
-    jaundice, malaria, tuberculosis, rheumatic fever...
-    heart disease, high or low blood pressure....

- allergy (asthma....)
- convulsions or diseases of the nervous system
- chronic disease (diabetes, malignancies, stomach ulcer)
- sexually transmitted disease

8. Have you previously been told not to give blood?

9. Do you have a hazardous occupation or hobby (ex: bus driving, diving...)?

Chapter 2: Blood collection

1. Premises for donor sessions

When sessions are performed by mobile teams, a realistic attitude towards environmental standards is necessary. The premises should satisfy common sense requirements for the health and safety of both the mobile teams and the donors concerned, with due regard to relevant legislation or regulations. Points to check should include adequate heating, lighting and ventilation, general cleanliness, provision of a secure supply of water and electricity, adequate sanitation, compliance with fire regulations, satisfactory access for unloading and loading of equipment by the mobile team, adequate space to allow free access to the bleed, and rest beds.

When the sessional venue is permanent and under the control of the transfusion centre, provision should additionally be made for proper cleaning by, for example, the use of non-slip, washable floor material installed without inaccessible corners, avoidance of internal window ledges, etc. Where possible, ventilation should be by an air-conditioning unit to avoid the need for open windows. Air changes, together with temperature and humidity control, should be adequate to cope with the maximum number of people likely to be in the room, and with the heat output from any equipment used. A maximum/minimum thermometer should be installed and checked daily by the quality control division.

2. Equipment used at blood donation sessions

Reference should be made to Chapter 21 for quality control procedures to be applied to equipment used at blood donation sessions.

3. Pre-donation checks

- The blood containers should be inspected before use for defects as well as after the donation. Defects may be hidden behind the label pasted on the container. The container should be inspected before use for the prescribed content (and appearance) of the anticoagulant solution. Abnormal moisture on the surface of the bag after unpacking will cause suspicion of leakage through a defect. If one or more bags in any package is found to be abnormally damp all the bags in the package should be rejected.

- Careful check must be made of the identity of the donor against the labels issued for that donation.

4. Preparation of the phlebotomy site

Although it is impossible to guarantee 100% sterility of the skin surface for phlebotomy, a strict, standardised procedure for the preparation of the phlebotomy area should exist. Of particular importance is that the antiseptic solution used be allowed to dry completely before venepuncture, The time taken will vary with the product used but should be subject to an absolute minimum of 30 seconds. The prepared area must not be touched with fingers before the needle has been inserted.

5. Need for successful venepuncture and proper mixing

The bleeding should be carried out in the following manner:

1. The needle should be inserted into the vein at first attempt. A second clean venepuncture with a new needle at a separate site is acceptable.

2. Proper mixing of the blood with the anti-coagulant should be guaranteed at all phases of the bleeding. To achieve this, one should pay attention to the following details:

   - as the blood begins to flow, it must immediately come into contact with the anticoagulant;

   - the flow of the blood must be sufficient and uninterrupted. Donation of a whole blood unit should ideally not last more than 10 minutes. If duration of the bleeding is longer than 12-15 minutes, the plasma should not be used for fractionation of labile plasma proteins or for the preparation of platelets.

     In the case of plasmapheresis, any interruption of the blood flow occurring during an apheresis procedure should exclude that donation from fractionation of labile plasma proteins or for the preparation of platelets.

   - when manual mixing is used, the blood bag must be inverted every 30-45 seconds. When an automated mixing is used, an appropriately validated system is required.

6.   Handling of filled containers and samples

Plastic containers should be checked after donation for any defect. During separation from the donor of the freshly filled plastic bag of blood, a completely efficient method of sealing the tube is obligatory. Immediately after sealing the donor tube, the contents of the part of the tube which still communicate with the bag should be completely discharged into the bag by stripping and the tube allowed to refill with mixed anticoagulated blood.

Alternatively, sampling could be done by transferring the needle directly from the vein into the rubber stopper of a sterile evacuated tube at the end of the donation. The blood is then sucked from the bag into the tube thus replacing the non-coagulated blood in the line by anticoagulated blood.

The organisation should be such as to minimise the possibility of errors in labelling of blood containers and blood samples, for example the taking of samples at the end of donation should be directly linked with the cessation of donation with the minimum possible time interval, and the blood bag and corresponding samples should not be removed from the donor's bedside until a satisfactory check on correct labelling has been carried out. In this respect, it is recommended that each bed should have its individual facilities for the handling of samples during donation and labelling.

7.   Special requirements

7.1   Apheresis

-       Separation and collection of blood components by cell-separators requires premises of suitable size, regular service and maintenance of the machines, and adequately trained personnel for operating such machines.

-       The donor should be observed closely during the procedure and a physician familiar with all aspects of apheresis must be available in order to provide assistance and emergency medical care procedures in case of adverse reaction.

-       Routine premedication of donors for the purpose of increasing component yield is not recommended.

-       The volume of extracorporeal blood should not exceed 13% of the donor's estimated blood volume.

7.2   Peripheral blood stem cells (PBSC)

The organisation for collection of PBSC shall have a director and a collection team of specifically trained personnel, otherwise collection of PBSC should meet the same criteria as for the selection of whole blood donors.

A written request to collect PBSC will be given to the collection physician and will contain the minimum cell count, volume or other surrogate marker of adequacy of collection.

Methods for collection shall employ aseptic technique and shall use procedures known to result in acceptable progenitor cell viability and recovery.

The cells collected should be packaged in a closed sterile container and labelled.

7.3   Cord Blood

The organisation for collection of umbilical cord blood shall have a director and a collection team of specifically trained personnel.

The cord blood collection service shall have a written agreement with the obstetrician regarding the collection of umbilical blood.

Collection protocols should be in a written form and comply with the standards of good medical practice.

Methods for collection shall employ aseptic technique and shall use procedures known to result in acceptable progenitor cell viability and recovery.

The cells collected should be packaged in a closed sterile container and labelled.

8.   Return of red blood cells of donors undergoing manual plasmapheresis

Since the biggest inherent danger in manual plasmapheresis is an interchange between two bags of concentrated red blood cells during their centrifugation and return to individual donors, a proper identification system to avoid this is an absolute necessity. For instance the donor may be asked to sign the label of the bag and to confirm his signature before the return of the red cells, though the ultimate responsibility lies with the individual carrying out this procedure.

In addition, use can be made of the integral numbering system on the pilot tube of plastic bags, perhaps by transferring this number to the wrist of the donor.

9. Storage of donor samples

The retention of donor samples for a period of time may provide useful scientific information. The provision of such systems is contingent on the availability of adequate human and financial resources.

10. Donor clinic documentation

Full records must be maintained at blood donation sessions, to cover the following parameters:

i.   the date, donation number and identity of the donor of each successful donation;

ii.   the date, donation number and identity of the donor for each unsuccessful donation, with reasons for the failure of the donation;

iii.   list of rejected donors with the reasons for their rejection;

iv.   full details of any adverse reactions in a donor at any stage of the procedure.

As far as possible the records of blood donation sessions should allow identification by blood transfusion staff of each important phase associated with the donation. These records should be used for the regular compilation of statistics which should be studied by the individual with ultimate responsibility for the blood donation session, who will take such action on them as deemed necessary.

Part C: Blood components

Chapter 3: Principles of component preparation

1.   Blood components - why should they be used?

Transfusion therapy in the past was largely dependent on the use of whole blood. While whole blood may still be used in certain limited circumstances, the thrust of modern transfusion therapy is to use the specific component that is clinically indicated. Components are those therapeutic constituents of blood that can be prepared by centrifugation filtration and freezing using conventional blood bank methodology.

Transfusions are used mainly for the following purposes:

-       to maintain blood volume;
-       to maintain oxygen transport;
-       to correct bleeding and coagulation disorders;
-       to correct an immunological deficiency;
-       to restore the lasting renewal of the cells of all haematopoietic lineages.

It is evident that one single product, whole blood, is not necessarily suitable for all these purposes unless the patient requiring treatment has multiple deficiencies. Even then, the storage defects of whole blood make it unsuitable for such replacement. Patients should be given the component needed to correct their specific deficiency. This will avoid unnecessary and possibly harmful infusion of surplus constituents. The change from collection of blood in glass bottles to multiple plastic bag systems has greatly facilitated the preparation of high quality components. Storage considerations are a major reason for promoting the use of components. Optimal conditions and consequently shelf life vary for different components. Red cells maintain functional capability best when refrigerated: hematopoietic progenitor cells (HPC) maintain their functions and effectiveness best when cryopreserved, the quality of plasma constituents is best maintained in the frozen state while it is now accepted that platelet storage is optimal when kept at room temperature with continuous agitation. Thus it is only the red cells whose storage requirement is fulfilled when whole blood is stored refrigerated, with consequent loss of therapeutic effectiveness of most of the other constituents.

Component therapy also offers logistic, ethical and economic advantages. In particular, plasma can be harvested in considerably increased quantities. The majority of patients requiring transfusion do not need the plasma in the whole unit and certainly not at a 1 to

1 ratio. Production of plasma derivatives can thus be facilitated by the use of red cells rather than whole blood.

2. Preparation procedure

Blood components may be prepared during collection using apheresis technology. Plasma, leucocytes and platelets may be obtained thus. Alternatively, whole blood may be collected in the traditional manner with the components being made available by the post-donation processing of whole blood. HPC may be harvested from bone marrow, peripheral blood or fetal blood by a combination of different techniques dependent on the source.

Due to the potential deterioration of activity and function of labile blood components, conditions of storage and time prior to processing are vital to the preparation of components. Delays in preparation or unsuitable conditions of storage may adversely affect quality of the final products.

3. Choice of anticoagulant and bag system

Whole blood is collected into a bag containing an anticoagulant solution. The solution contains citrate and cell nutrients such as glucose and adenine. The first centrifugation steps will remove about half of these nutrients from the residual red cells. Thus it may be more logical to provide the proper nutrients for the cells using a resuspension medium instead of incorporating them in the initial anticoagulant solution. HPC are collected in an anticoagulant solution either containing citrate or heparin; nutrients like glucose may be present in the anticoagulant solution to bridge the storage period between collection and cryopreservation.

In order to maintain a closed system throughout the separation procedure, a multiple bag configuration, either ready made or sterile-docked, should be used. The design and arrangement of the pack system should be such as to permit the required sterile preparation of the desired component.

Although only use of closed systems is recommended for all steps in component processing, open systems may sometimes be necessary due to local constraints in an environment specifically designed to minimise the risk of bacterial contamination. When open systems are employed, careful attention should be given to use of sterile procedures. The products so prepared should be transfused within 24 hours of processing, if processed and stored at 4 °C, or within 6 hours of processing if stored at room temperature.

4. Principles of centrifugation

The sedimentation behaviour of blood cells is determined by their size as well as the difference of their density from that of the surrounding fluid (See Table 1). Other factors are viscosity of the medium and flexibility of the cells which are temperature dependent. The optimal temperature with respect to these factors is 20 °C or higher.

Table 1:   Volume and density of principal blood constituents

	Mean Density (g/mL)	Mean Volume 10^{-15} litre
Plasma	1.026	
Platelets	1.058	16
Monocytes	1.062	740
Lymphocytes	1.070	230
Neutrophils	1.082	270
Red Cells	1.100	87

In the first phase of centrifugation, the surrounding fluid is only a mixture of plasma and anticoagulant solution. Leucocytes and red cells now sediment more rapidly than platelets as they both have a bigger volume than platelets. In a later phase, depending on the time and speed of centrifugation, most of the leucocytes and red cells therefore settle in the lower half of the bag and the upper half contains platelet rich plasma. More prolonged centrifugation results in platelet sedimentation driven by a force proportional to the square of the number of rotations per minute and the distance of each cell to the centre of the rotor, whereas the leucocytes being now surrounded by a fluid of higher density (the red cell mass) move upwards. At the end of centrifugation, cell-free plasma is in the upper part of the bag and red cells at the bottom. Platelets accumulate on top of the red cell layer while the majority of leucocytes are to be found immediately below in the top 10 mL of red cell mass. Haematopoietic progenitor cells have similar characteristics to normal mononuclear blood cells. However their contaminants may be immature or malignant cells from different haematopoietic lineages which commonly have larger sizes and lower densities than their mature counterparts.

The choice to be made is the speed and time of centrifugation which will determine the composition of the desired component, i.e. if platelet-rich plasma is desired, centrifugation should stop prior to the phase where platelet sedimentation commences. A low centrifugation speed will allow for some variation in centrifugation time. If cell-free plasma is required, fast centrifugation for an adequate time will allow separation to cell-poor plasma and densely packed cells. It is important that the optimal conditions for a good separation be carefully standardised for each centrifuge. A number of choices exist for the selection of a procedure for centrifugation for component preparation from whole blood.

Table 2 outlines four different methods of performing the first step in the separation of whole blood as well as the approximate composition of the resulting initial components.

The choice of the initial separation step strongly influences the methods of further processing of the initial fractions. This leads to a system of interdependent methodologies for the preparation of a set of final products. Whenever a method for the preparation of a blood component is specified, reference should always be made to the initial separation step.

5.   Separation

5.1.   Separation after the initial centrifugation

After centrifugation, the bag system is carefully removed from the centrifuge. The primary bag is placed into a plasma extraction system and the layers are transferred, one by one, into satellite bags within the closed system.

The choice to be made is whether or not the buffy coat is to be removed from the packed cells into a separate bag. The advantage of this is that the remaining red cells are leucocyte-poor and will remain aggregate-poor during storage.

For an estimation of the results that can be obtained using the four options, see Table 2.

Dependent on the choice of technique for component preparation:

methods I and II will be followed by recentrifugation of the platelet-rich plasma for the preparation of cell-free plasma and platelet concentrate;

method III will be followed by preparation of platelet concentrate from buffy coats.

Table 2:   Four different methods of initial separation of whole blood and the approximate composition of the fractions obtained (figures refer to a standard donation of 450 mL ± 10% taken into 60-70 mL of anticoagulant)

Method	I	II	III	IV
Centrifugation speed	low	low	high	high
Separation into	plasma + buffy coat + red cells	plasma + red cells	plasma + buffy coat + red cells	plasma + red cells
Resulting crude fractions Plasma, volume platelets, leucocytes	200-280 mL 70-80% 5-10%	200-280 mL 70-80% 5-10%	270-320 mL 10-20% 2-5%	270-330 mL 10-20% 2-5%
	75-80% 5-15% 25-45%	65-75% 20-30% 90-95%	85-90% 10-20% 25-45%	80-90% 80-90% 95-98%
Red cells, EVF* platelets leucocytes	50-70% 10-15% 10-25% 60-70%		40-60% 10-15% 80-90% 50-70%	
Buffy coat, EVF* red cells platelets leucocytes				

*   Erythrocyte or cellular volume fraction

The advantage of the removal of buffy coat is that the remaining red cells can be resuspended into a solution designed to offer optimal conditions for red cell storage, e.g. SAGM. The resuspension may still be done within the closed system. Cell-free plasma can now be frozen and be stored as fresh frozen plasma to be used as such or as a starting material for further products.

5.2 Other separation principles

- ### Zonal centrifugation

Sedimentation of blood cells can be achieved when a centrifugal force is exerted on flowing blood more or less perpendicular to the direction of the flow. The efficiency of the separation depends on the ratio between the centrifugal force and the flow velocity. At a high ratio the plasma obtained is platelet-poor, and at a lower ratio platelet-rich plasma can be obtained.

A number of apheresis devices are available in which this principle is applied for the production of cell-poor plasma or platelet-rich plasma.

A further application of zonal centrifugation is the removal of plasma protein from a red cell suspension. A unit of red cells is introduced into the centrifuge bowl, a flow of washing fluid is then maintained until the protein concentration in the effluent is sufficiently reduced. Centrifugation is discontinued and the "washed" blood cell suspension is harvested.

The same principle is also used for both the addition and the removal of cryoprotectant before freezing and after thawing of blood cell suspensions in cryopreservation.

- ### Buoyant density centrifugation

Buoyant density centrifugation of blood, bone marrow or buffycoat cells on top of a layer with a density of 1.077 g/mL leads to a layer of mononuclear cells floating on the interface and a pellet of red cells and granulocytes which have penetrated through the separating medium according to the density of the cells involved.

Buoyant density separation is generally applicable for separations based on density differences between cells e.g. also for the separation of cells complexed with red cells to rosettes from the non-rosetted cells.

- ### Counter current centrifugation (elutriation)

Counter current centrifugation enables the separation of cells according to their size. The principle is based upon the ability to pump a suspension of cells through a chamber in the rotor of a centrifuge in the direction opposite to the centrifugal force, during the run of the centrifuge. In this system mononuclear cells can be collected in the chamber, depleted of platelets, granulocytes and red cells.

Counter current centrifugation is also applicable for the separation of cells rosetted with red cells from non-rosetted cells.

- ### Filtration

At present, two major types of filtration are available for blood component preparation:

-    the separation of plasma from blood by cross-flow filtration;

-       the removal of leucocytes from cell suspensions by depth-filtration.

i.   Cross-flow filtration

When blood flows along a membrane with a pore size allowing free passage of plasma proteins but not of blood cells, cell-free plasma may be obtained by filtration.

Plasmapheresis devices have been developed in which a pumping system takes blood from the donor's vein, mixes it at a constant ratio with anti-coagulant solution and then leads it along a plasma-permeable membrane (flat membrane or hollow fibre system). Two pressures are exerted on the blood: one parallel to the membrane, keeping the blood flowing along the membrane, and the other perpendicular to the membrane, the actual filtration pressure. This system prevents accumulation of cells on the membrane while plasma is removed from the blood (the haematocrit in the system may increase from 40% to 75%). In some devices, velocity of the flow parallel to the membrane is increased by an additional vortex action or by movement of the membrane.

When a specified extra-corporeal cell volume has been reached, the cells are reinfused to the donor, and the next cycle starts until the required volume of cell-free plasma has been obtained.

ii.   Depth filtration

Owing the specific properties of platelets and granulocytes as well as the low flexibility of lymphocytes, these cells are more easily trapped in a filter bed of fibres than red cells. Three mechanisms of trapping have been recognised in filters used for leucocyte depletion of red cell concentrates:

a)   the activation of platelets leading to the attachment of these cells to the fibres in the top of the filter, followed by the interaction of the attached platelets and granulocytes;

b)   the activation of granulocytes by another type of fibre leading to attachment of these cells in the middle part of the filter;

c)   the obstruction of the lymphocytes in the pores and fork junctions of the finest fibre material in the bottom layers of the filter. Blow-moulded mats of fibre material with different pore sizes and fibre thicknesses are now used to produce leucocyte depletion filters for red cell concentrates.

        Surface treatment of the filter material may prevent activation of platelets and now allows the production of filters which reduce the contaminating leucocytes from platelet concentrates by sieving only.

        Filters used for leucocyte removal from red cells or platelets show considerable variations in efficacy and capacity. Besides filter properties, the final result of filtration is influenced by several process parameters (e.g., flow rate, temperature, priming and rinsing) and properties of the component to be filtered (e.g., storage history of the component, number of leucocytes and number of platelets). When a standardised filtration procedure is established, limits must therefore be set for all the variables affecting the efficacy of filtration and the Standard Operating Procedures (SOP's) should be fully validated under the condition to be used.

-       Immune adsorbent techniques

The specific isolation of particular type of mononuclear cells during the preparation of stem cells often makes use of immune adsorbent techniques. Two types of procedures are used, either the specific removal of cells contaminating the stem cell preparation ("negative selection") or the isolation of HPC ("positive selection").

Different monoclonal antibodies are applied in the following techniques: immune rosette formation, magnetic beads or biotinylated beads used for these purposes.

The systems to be used during the consecutive steps of the HPC preparation should be designed in such a way that cell losses in dead spaces of tubes, column, chambers, and bags are reduced to a minimum.

-       Washing of cellular components

This technique is occasionally used when there is requirement for protein free cells.

6.   Cryoprecipitation

The isolation of some plasma proteins, most importantly Factor VIII, fibronectin and fibrinogen, can be achieved by making use of their reduced solubility at low temperature. In practice, this is done by freezing units of plasma, thawing and centrifugation at low temperature.

7.   Freezing and thawing of plasma

7.1   Rationale

Freezing is a critical step in the conservation of plasma Factor VIII. During freezing, pure ice is formed and the plasma solutes are concentrated in the remaining water. When the solubility of the solutes is exceeded, each solute forms crystals but may be influenced by the used anticoagulants. Further studies on this aspect are ongoing.

The ice formation depends on the rate of heat extraction, whereas the diffusion rates of the solutes determine their displacement. At slow freezing rates, the diffusion of solutes copes with the rate of ice formation; solutes are increasingly concentrated in the middle of a plasma unit.

Since all solutes are displaced simultaneously, the Factor VIII molecules are exposed to a high concentration of salts for a prolonged time and thus inactivated. At a high freezing rate, the ice formation overtakes the solute displacement and small clusters of solidified solute are homogeneously trapped in the ice without prolonged contact between highly concentrated salts and Factor VIII.

To achieve the highest yield of Factor VIII, citrated plasma should be frozen to -30 °C or below.

Decrease of Factor VIII during freezing occurs when the solidification of plasma takes more than one hour. This can be monitored by measuring the total protein content of a core sample of the frozen plasma; this protein concentration should be identical with the total protein content of plasma before freezing. An optimal freezing rate is obtainable when a heat extraction of 38 kcal per hour per unit of plasma is achieved, and can be monitored by the use of thermocouples.

In order to effectively incorporate these techniques into a coherent daily routine, the blood bank staff has to be familiar with the thinking behind the technique as well as its potential limitations and pitfalls.

7.2   Methods of freezing

When freezing citrated plasma, the rate of cooling must be as rapid as possible and ideally should bring the core temperature down to -30 °C or below within 60 minutes. If this is not possible, the minimum acceptable rate of freezing should bring the core temperature down to -30 °C within 4 hours.

Experience has shown that it sometimes takes several hours in an environmental temperature of -30 °C and heat transfer by air. The time must be reduced to less than one hour and if possible, less than half an hour, for example by the following means:

-    plasma should be presented in a regular configuration to maximise exposure to the freezing process (e.g. bags laid flat or in formers if vertical);

-    immersion in an environment at very low temperature;

-    if a liquid environment is used, it should have been shown that the container cannot be penetrated by the solvent.

8.   The use of an open system and devices for sterile connections

It is suggested that any new development in component preparation involving an open system should be subjected to intensive testing during the developmental phase for maintenance of sterility.

Other than this, routine sterility testing as an ongoing quality control measure is thought to be of limited value. Blood components prepared by an open system should be used as quickly as possible.

Components prepared in systems using fully validated sterile connecting devices may be stored as if prepared in a closed system.

9.   Additional procedures

9.1   Blood products treated with ionising radiation

Viable lymphocytes in blood products can cause fatal graft-versus-host reaction in severely immuno-compromised patients, e.g. transplant recipients and children with severe immuno-deficiency syndromes. Other categories of patients are also at risk of this rare complication e.g. following intrauterine transfusion, transfusion between family members and transfusion of HLA- matched components.

Lymphocytes can be rendered non-viable by exposure to ionising radiation. This treatment does not cause significant harm to other blood components and an irradiated component can therefore safely be given to all patients.

An irradiation dose of 25 to 40 Gray is usually considered sufficient. Exposure time must be standardised for each irradiation source and also adjusted at suitable intervals.

Red cell products may be irradiated up to 14 days after collection and thereafter stored until the 28th day after collection. In view of the increased potassium leak from red cells consequent to their irradiation, such cells intended for intrauterine or neonatal transfusion should be used within 48 hours of irradiation.

The use of radiation-sensitive labels to demonstrate that the component has been irradiated is recommended.

9.2   Cytomegalovirus-free blood components

Cytomegalovirus (CMV) is a common infectious agent that can be transmitted by transfusion of blood components. The risk of disease transmission is highest with fresh products containing mono- and polynuclear white cells. CMV infection is often asymptomatic in healthy persons. Antibodies usually appear 4 to 8 weeks after infection and can be demonstrated in standard screening tests. Since the infection is common, the test has to be repeated on each donation from a previously sero-negative donor.

Infection caused by this virus is usually not clinically significant in immuno-competent recipients, but can cause severe, even fatal, disease in certain patients not previously exposed to the virus:

-    transplant recipients,
-    patients with severe immuno-deficiency,
-    foetus in utero,
-    low weight premature infants and neonates.

These patients should receive components from anti-CMV negative donors as should anti-CMV negative pregnant women, to protect the foetus. The use of leucocyte-depleted components is an acceptable alternative.

10. Definitions and minimum requirements

Since blood components are used to correct a known deficit, each preparation must be subjected to strict quality control. The aim is to produce "pure" components, but a very high degree of purity can be difficult and expensive to obtain and might not even be necessary in all instances. However, it is absolutely necessary to declare the quality and to be able to make different types of preparations in order to give the clinicians a reasonable choice for patients with different transfusion demands.

For example, a red cell concentrate can be produced with varying concentrations of contaminating white cells and platelets. A buffy coat depleted preparation where > 70% of the white cells and > 90% of the platelets have been removed is useful to the majority of recipients since microaggregate formation during storage will be inhibited. If the patient has antibodies against leucocyte antigens or if it can be foreseen that he/she will need a very large number of transfusions, white cell depletion must be much more efficient.

In order to institute an adequate scheme of component therapy, all products must be carefully defined and minimum requirements set. Clinical users should be informed of the properties of all components.

11. Introducing component preparation in a blood bank

Laboratories with little or no experience of component preparation should allow their staff to attend training courses and visit blood banks with extensive experience of work of this type.

Equipment should be purchased with provision for adequate service and maintenance of the machines. A method must be chosen which will achieve the desired results. All steps in the procedure should be clearly explained in a manual which should be available at the work bench.

Before the method is taken into routine use, it must be fully validated and a Standard Operating Procedure (SOP) established. Each prepared unit must be carefully checked until it is verified that the intended quality is obtained. Routinely prepared products should then be subjected to regular quality control.

12. Product control - quality assurance

In all respects the preparation of blood products and components should follow the principles of Good Manufacturing Practice (GMP).

The purpose of product control is to help the blood bank maintain a high and even quality of the prepared product. In this way, clinical outcome will improve, confidence in component therapy will increase and the introduction of an adequate component therapy programme will be facilitated.

Lack of accuracy, deviation from SOP or incorrect handling when blood is processed will not give the intended component quality.

Method descriptions and product control go hand in hand; therefore an SOP for product control is also necessary. The results of product control must be continuously evaluated and steps taken to correct defective procedures or equipment.

In the following chapters, the different blood components will be defined and described. Principles of good preparation methods, storage and transport will also be described, and finally guidelines for quality control will be given.

13.   Storage of blood components

Storage conditions for blood components must be designed to preserve optimal viability and function during the whole storage period. The risk of bacterial contamination decreases substantially if only closed separation and storage systems are used. Storage routines must also be controlled continuously, as should issue and return routines; transport of blood components must also take place in a safe and controlled way.

13.1   Equipment

Blood components are stored at 22 °C, at 2 °C to 6 °C or at different temperatures below 0 °C. Whatever type of storage device is chosen, the following points should be considered before purchase:

i.   Refrigerators and freezers must have surplus capacity. The space should be easy to inspect.

ii.   The operation must be reliable and temperature distribution must be uniform within the unit.

iii.   The equipment must have temperature recording and alarm devices.

iv.   The equipment should be easy to clean and should withstand strong detergents. It should also conform to local safety requirements.

13.2   Storage at 2 °C to 6 °C

Refrigerators for blood component storage should be restricted to whole blood, blood components, pilot tubes and test reagents.

Separate space should be reserved for:

-       units for issue,

-       units selected for certain patients including autologous donations,

-       units kept in quarantine awaiting completion of testing,

-       outdated and discarded units.

The space for each of these component types should be clearly indicated. The temperature within the unit should be recorded continuously. The sensor of the thermograph should be placed within a blood bag filled with 10% glycerol solution to a volume of 250 mL or a volume equivalent to the normal volume of the stored component. This container should be placed in the upper part of the refrigerated space. In large refrigerated rooms, two such sensors should be applied.

The alarm system should preferably have both acoustic and optical signals and should be tested regularly.

Refrigerators for blood components should ideally be connected to a reserve power unit as well as the main supply.

13.3   Storage of frozen plasma components

The eutectic point of plasma is -23 °C. To allow for temperature fluctuation during use, a transfusion centre should have a freezer routinely capable of running at -30 °C or below.

The freezers may also contain non-therapeutic plasma and serum products. Separate space should be allocated for the different types of products and be clearly marked to avoid mistakes.

Freezers with automatic defrosting should be avoided unless it can be guaranteed that the low temperature is maintained during defrosting.

The temperature within the freezer should be recorded continuously. The alarm system should preferably have both acoustic and optical signals, and should be tested regularly.

Freezers should ideally be connected to a reserve power source as well as the main supply.

13.4   Storage at 22 °C

Platelets are stored at room temperature (22 °C ± 2 °C). A closed device that permits temperature control is recommended. If such a device is unavailable, the space chosen should be capable of maintaining the required constant temperature.

The platelets should be stored in agitators which should:

-        enable satisfactory mixing in the bag as well as gas exchange through the wall of the bag;

-        avoid folding of the bags;

-        have a set speed to avoid foaming.

A closed device should have thermograph and alarm systems. Otherwise, a control thermometer should be used at the storage site and checked several times daily. The speed of the agitator should be tested regularly according to the manufacturer's recommendations.

The anticoagulant solutions used in blood collection have been developed to prevent coagulation and to permit storage of red cells for a certain period of time. While originally designed for whole blood storage, they have also been used in blood from which components are prepared. All of the solutions contain sodium citrate, citric acid and glucose, some of them in addition to adenine, guanosine and phosphate.

Citrate binds calcium and prevents clotting of the blood. Glucose is used by the red cell during storage and each glucose molecule gives two molecules of adenosine tri-phosphate (ATP) which is formed by phosphorylation of adenosine di-phosphate (ADP). ATP is an energy-rich molecule which is used to support the energy-demanding functions of the erythrocyte, such as membrane flexibility and certain membrane transport functions. During its action in energy-consuming operations, ATP is transferred back to ADP. Citric acid is added to the anticoagulant in order to obtain a hydrogen ion concentration which is suitably high at the beginning of storage at +4 °C. Without this addition the blood would be too alkaline at storage temperature. During storage, an increasing acidity occurs which reduces glycolysis. The content of adenosine nucleotides (ATP, ADP, AMP) decreases during storage. By addition of adenine which is a main component in the adenosine nucleotides, the erythrocytes can synthesise new AMP, ADP and ATP and compensate for (or reduce) the losses.

When red cell concentrates are prepared, a considerable part of the glucose and adenine is removed with the plasma. If not compensated for in other ways (e.g. larger amount than normal of adenine and glucose in the anticoagulant or by separate addition of a suspension/preservative medium), sufficient viability of the red cells can only be maintained if the cells are not over-concentrated. Normal CPD-adenine red cell concentrate should therefore not have an EVF above 0.70. This also keeps the viscosity sufficiently low to permit transfusion of the concentrate without pre-administration dilution.

Platelets and leucocytes rapidly lose their viability at 4 °C. They form microaggregates which are present in considerable amounts even after 3 to 4 days' storage of whole blood and even more so in red cell concentrates. Microaggregates can pass through the filters of ordinary blood transfusion sets. They are considered to be able to cause decreased lung function by blocking the lung capillaries and this may be of clinical importance in massive transfusions. Removal of platelets during component preparation reduces microaggregate formation. Likewise, leucocyte depletion by buffy coat removal will also reduce the frequency of febrile transfusion reactions and will help in obtaining high-grade depletion of leucocytes when leucocyte-removal filters are used for this purpose.

The use of an additive or suspension medium allows maintenance of red cell viability even if more than 90% of the plasma is removed. The use of sodium chloride, adenine and glucose is necessary for viability while other sugars are used to further stabilise the cell membrane and prevent haemolysis.

13.6 Erythrocyte preparations

Red cells may be stored in the fluid state at a controlled temperature of 2 °C to 6 °C. The performance of the storage refrigerator must itself be carefully controlled (see Chapter 21).

The maximum duration of storage (expiry date) should be noted on each container. This duration may vary with the type of preparation (concentration of cells, formula of anticoagulant, use of additive suspension fluid, etc.) and should be determined for each type on the basis of achieving a mean 24 hour post-transfusion survival of no less than 75% of the transfused red cells.

Red cells in the frozen state should be prepared and reconstituted according to an approved protocol, be stored at -80 °C or below, and produce satisfactory post-transfusion survival figures.

13.7 Platelet storage

Platelet preparations are particularly influenced by storage conditions. Platelet metabolism, and consequently post-transfusion function and viability, is dependent especially on adequate oxygen availability, the temperature and the pH of the suspending solution. Accordingly, the use of special gas-permeable plastic containers, proper temperature (20 °C - 24 °C) and adequate agitation during storage are all features necessary for proper storage of this component.

13.8 Granulocyte preparations

Ordinarily, granulocyte suspensions are prepared for a specific patient and administered immediately. If intermediate storage is unavoidable this should be at a controlled 22 °C ± 2 °C for a maximum of 24 hours.

13.9 Plasma components

Recommended storage conditions for fresh frozen plasma and cryoprecipitate and for cryoprecipitate-depleted plasma are given in Table 3.

Table 3: Recommended storage conditions

Product	Temperature and length of storage
Fresh frozen plasma and cryoprecipitate	24 months at -40 °C or below 12 months at -30 °C to -40 °C 6 months at -25 °C to -30 °C 3 months at -18 °C to -25 °C
Cryoprecipitate-depleted plasma	2 years at -18 °C or below

14.   Issue and transportation

Blood components should be transported by a system that will maintain the recommended storage temperature of the component. The containers used in transport should be well insulated, easy to clean and easy to handle. Where a dedicated refrigerated vehicle is used the principles applying to control of the refrigerators should be observed. Alternatively, systems for road or rail transport using controlled cooling elements may be considered. These coolants must not come into close contact with the blood bags. If the blood is to be transported over long distances or if the ambient temperature is high, the volume of the cooling elements to blood bags should be 2:1.

Red cell products must be kept between +2 °C and +10 °C; and platelet products between +22 °C and +24 °C. Frozen plasma should be transported in the frozen state as close as possible to the recommended storage temperature.

It is recommended that some form of temperature indicator be used to monitor the in-transit temperature. On receipt, if not intended for immediate transfusion, the product should be transferred to storage under recommended conditions.

The temperature on receipt can be monitored as follows:

> Take 2 bags from the container, place a thermometer between the bags and fix them together with rubber bands. Quickly replace them into the container and close the lid. Read the temperature after 5 minutes. The temperature of red cell bags should not go below +1 °C nor exceed 10 °C. Alternatively an electronic sensing device may be used to take immediate measure from the surface of a pack.

Returned blood components should not be reissued for transfusion if the bag has been penetrated or entered, the product not maintained continuously within the approved temperature range or if there is evidence of leakage, abnormal colour change or excess haemolysis. The proper identification, time of issue and transit history should be fully documented.

Chapter 4: Whole blood

Definition

Whole blood for transfusion is blood taken from a suitable donor using a sterile and pyrogen-free anticoagulant and container. The major use of whole blood is as source material for blood component preparation.

Properties

Freshly drawn whole blood maintains all its properties for a limited period of time. Rapid deterioration of Factor VIII, leucocytes and platelets makes whole blood an unsuitable product for treatment of haemostatic disturbances when stored beyond the first 24 hours. Upon further liquid storage a number of changes occur, such as increase of oxygen affinity and loss of viability of the red cells, loss of coagulation factor activity (Factors VIII and V), loss of platelet viability and function, formation of microaggregates, release of intracellular components such as potassium and leucocyte proteases, and activation of plasma factors such as kallikrein.

Methods of preparation

1.   Pre-donation checks

-    The blood containers should be inspected before use for defects as well as after the donation. Defects may be hidden behind the label pasted on the container. The container should be inspected before use for the prescribed content (and appearance) of the anticoagulant solution. Abnormal moisture on the surface of the bag after unpacking will cause suspicion of leakage through a defect. If one or more bags in any package is found to be abnormally damp all the bags in the package should be rejected.

-    A careful check must be made of the identity of the donor against the labels issued for that donation.

2.   Preparation of the phlebotomy site

Although it is impossible to guarantee 100% sterility of the skin surface for phlebotomy, a strict, standardised procedure for the preparation of the phlebotomy area should exist. Of particular importance is that the antiseptic solution used be allowed to dry completely before venepuncture, The time taken will vary with the product used but should be subject to an absolute minimum of 30 seconds. The prepared area must not be touched with fingers before the needle has been inserted.

3. Need for successful venepuncture and proper mixing

The bleeding should be carried out in the following manner:

i.   The needle should be inserted into the vein at first attempt. A second clean venipuncture with a new needle at a separate site is acceptable.

ii.   Proper mixing of the blood with the anti-coagulant should be guaranteed at all phases of the bleeding. To achieve this, one should pay attention to the following details:

-       As the blood begins to flow, it must immediately come into contact with the anticoagulant.

-       The flow of the blood must be sufficient and constant. Donation of a whole blood unit should ideally not last more than 10 minutes. If duration of the bleeding is longer than 12-15 minutes, the plasma should not be used for fractionation of labile plasma proteins as for the preparation of platelets.

-       When manual mixing is used, the blood bag must be inverted every 30-45 seconds. When an automated mixing is used, appropriately validated system is required.

4. Handling of filled containers and samples

Plastic containers should be checked after donation for any defect which may be revealed after filling. During separation from the donor of the freshly filled plastic bag of blood, a completely efficient method of sealing the tube is obligatory. Immediately after sealing the donor tube, the contents of the part of the tube which still communicate with the bag should be completely discharged into the bag by stripping and the tube allowed to refill with mixed anticoagulated blood.

Alternatively, sampling could be done by transferring the needle directly from the vein into the rubber stopper of a sterile evacuated tube at the end of the donation. The blood is then sucked from the bag into the tube thus replacing the non-coagulated blood in the line by anticoagulated blood.

The organisation should be such as to minimise the possibility of errors in labelling of blood containers and blood samples, for example the taking of samples at the end of donation should be directly linked with the cessation of donation with the minimum possible time interval, and the blood bag and corresponding samples should not be removed from the donor's bedside until a satisfactory check on correct labelling has been carried out. In this respect, it is recommended that each bed should have its individual facilities for the handling of samples during donation and labelling.

5. Maintenance of records

Full records must be maintained at blood donation sessions, to cover the following parameters:

i.   the date, donation number and identity of the donor of each successful donation;

ii.   the date, donation number and identity of the donor for each unsuccessful donation, with reasons for the failure of the donation;

iii.   full details of rejected donors with the reasons for their rejection;

iv.   full details of any adverse reactions in a donor at any stage of the procedure.

So far as possible, the records of blood donation sessions should allow identification by blood transfusion staff of each important phase associated with the donation. These records should be used for regular compilation of statistics which should be studied by the individual with ultimate responsibility for the blood donation session, who will take such action on them as deemed necessary.

Labelling

The labelling should comply with the relevant national legislation and international agreements. The label on the container states:

-    the name and the volume of the preparation;

-    the producer's name and address (clear text or code);

-    the donation number;

-    the ABO group;

-    the Rh (D) group, specifying "Rh (D) positive" if D positive or "Rh (D) negative" if D negative;

-    the composition and volume of the anticoagulant solution;

-    the date of collection and expiry date;

-    the temperature of storage;

-    that the blood must not be used for transfusion if there is abnormal haemolysis or other deterioration;

-    that the blood must be administered through a 170-200 μm filter.

Storage and stability

Donations intended for transfusion as whole blood shall be stored at 2 °C to 6 °C. The storage time depends on the anticoagulant/preservative solution used. For CPD-A 1 the storage time is 35 days.

Microaggregates are formed on storage.

During storage there is a progressive decrease in the labile coagulation factors V and VIII, an increase in potassium and acidity in the plasma and a rapid decrease in platelet viability because of storage at 2 °C to 6 °C.

The oxygen-carrying capacity decreases during storage due to progressive loss of 2,3 bis-phosphoglycerate (2,3 BPG, previous name 2,3 di-phosphoglycerate DPG). After 10 days of storage in CPD-A 1 all 2,3 BPG is lost. However, it regenerates after transfusion in the circulation of the recipient.

Quality assurance

Much of the quality control necessary to ensure the safety and efficacy of whole blood takes place at the time of blood collection. In addition to the measures carried out at the time of collection, the parameters listed in Table 4 must also be checked.

Table 4   Tests to be carried out on whole blood donation

Parameter to be checked	Quality requirement	Frequency of control	Control executed by
ABO, Rh (D)	grouping	all units	grouping lab
HIV-Abs	negative by approved screening test	all units	screening lab
HBsAg	negative by approved screening test	all units	screening lab
ALT (when required)	not elevated (as specified by national authorities)	all units	screening lab
HBc-Ab (when required)	negative by approved screening test	all units	screening lab
HCV-Ab	negative by approved screening test	all units	screening lab
Syphilis (when required)	negative by screening test	all units	screening lab
CMV-Ab (when required)	negative by screening test	as required	screening lab
HTLV-Abs (when required)	negative by screening test	all units	screening lab
Standard donation	450 mL ± 10% volume excluding anticoagulant Other volumes according to national regulations	weighing of 1% of all units	processing lab

Transport

After collection, blood should be kept at a controlled temperature , usually between 2 °C and 10 °C. If whole blood is to be used for platelet preparation, the bag should be kept on a cooling device at about 20 °C.

Indications for use

Where component preparation is routine, whole blood must be considered as a source material and has no, or only a very restricted, place in transfusion practice. In the absence of appropriate plasma substitutes and blood components, the use of whole blood can only be envisaged in clinical settings where red cell and blood volume deficit are simultaneously present.

Precautions in use

Compatibility of whole blood with the intended recipient must be verified by suitable pre-transfusion testing.

Consideration should be given to the use of a microaggregate filter.

Whole blood is contra-indicated in:

- anaemia without blood volume loss;

- various types of plasma intolerance;

- intolerance due to alloimmunisation against leucocyte antigens.

Side-effects

- Circulatory overload.

- Haemolytic transfusion reactions.

- Non-haemolytic transfusion reaction (mainly chills, fever and urticaria).

- Sepsis by inadvertent bacterial contamination of blood.

- Syphilis can be transmitted when whole blood has been stored for less than 96 hours at 4 °C.

- Viral transmission (hepatitis, HIV, etc.) is possible despite careful donor selection and screening procedures.

- Protozoal transmission (e.g. malaria) may occur in rare instances.

- Alloimmunisation against HLA and red cell antigens.

- Citrate intoxication in neonates and in patients with impaired liver function.

- Biochemical imbalance in massive transfusion, e.g. hyperkalaemia.

- Post-transfusion purpura.

- Transfusion related acute lung injury.

Chapter 5: Red cells

Definition

A component obtained by removal of part of the plasma from whole blood, without further processing.

Properties

The erythrocyte volume fraction (EVF) of the component is 0.65-0.75; Each unit should have a minimum of 45 g of haemoglobin at the end of processing.

The unit contains all of the original unit's red cells. The greater part of its leucocytes (about 2.5 to 3.0×10^9 cells) and a varying content of platelets depending on the method of centrifugation are retained, no effort having been made for removal.

Methods of preparation

For the preparation of the component, removal of the plasma from the whole blood unit after centrifugation, or spontaneous sedimentation, is performed.

Labelling

The labelling should comply with the relevant national legislation and international agreements. The label on the container states:

- the name and the volume of the component;

- the producer's name and address (clear text or code);

- the donation number;

- the ABO group;

- the Rh (D) group, specifying "Rh (D)-positive" if D positive or "Rh (D)-negative" if D negative;

- the composition and volume of the anticoagulant solution;

- the date of collection and expiry date;

- the temperature of storage;

- that the component must not be used for transfusion if there is abnormal haemolysis or other deterioration;

- that the component must be administered through a 170-200 μm filter.

Storage and stability

As for whole blood. Microaggregates are formed on storage.

Quality assurance

As for whole blood with the exceptions indicated in Table 5.

Table 5: Quality asurance

Parameter to be checked	Quality requirement (specification)	Frequency of control	Control executed by
Volume	280 ± 50 mL	1% of all units	Processing lab
EVF	0.65 to 0.75	4 units per month	QC lab
Haemoglobin	minimum 45 g/unit	4 units per month	QC lab
Haemolysis at the end of storage	<0.8% of red cell masses	4 units per month	QC lab

Transport

Transport by a non-refrigerated vehicle requires a cooled and insulated container.

Indications for use

Red cells are used for replacement in blood loss and for the therapy of anaemia.

Precautions in use

Compatibility of red cells with the intended recipient must be verified by suitable pre-transfusion testing.

Consideration should be given to the use of a microaggregate filter.

Red cells are not recommended in:

- various types of plasma intolerance;

- intolerance due to alloimmunisation against leucocyte antigens;

- exchange transfusion in newborns unless supplementary plasma is added;

- transfusion in premature infants and recipients with a risk of iron overload, unless used within 14 days of donation to reduce frequency of transfusion.

Side-effects

- Circulatory overload.

- Haemolytic transfusion reaction.

- Non-haemolytic transfusion reaction (mainly chills, fever).

- Alloimmunisation against HLA and red cell antigens.

- Syphilis can be transmitted when red cells have been stored for less than 96 hours at 4 °C.

- Viral transmission (hepatitis, HIV, etc.) is possible despite careful donor selection and screening procedures.

- Protozoal transmission (e.g. malaria) may occur in rare instances.

- Sepsis due to inadvertent bacterial contamination.

- Biochemical imbalance in massive transfusion, e.g. hyperkalaemia.

- Post-transfusion purpura.

- Transfusion related acute lung injury

Chapter 6: Red cells, buffy coat removed (red cells: BCR)

Definition

A component prepared by removal of part of the plasma and the buffy-coat layer from whole blood.

Properties

The EVF of the component is 0.65 to 0.75.

The unit contains all, except 20 to 30 mL, of the original unit's red cells. Each unit should have a minimum haemoglobin content of 43 g.

The leucocyte content is less than 1.2×10^9 cells per unit and the average platelet content less than 10×10^9 cells per unit.

Methods of preparation

For the preparation of the component, the plasma and 40 to 60 mL of the buffy coat layer are removed from the whole blood unit after centrifugation or sedimentation. Sufficient plasma is returned to the red cell unit to give EVF 0.65 to 0.75.

Labelling

The labelling should comply with the relevant national legislation and international agreements. The label on the container states:

-   the name and the volume of the component;

-   the producer's name and address (clear text or code);

-   the donation number;

-   the ABO group;

-   the Rh (D) group, specifying "Rh (D)-positive" if D positive or "Rh (D)-negative" if D negative;

-   the composition and volume of the anticoagulant solution;

-   the date of collection and expiry date;

-   the temperature of storage;

- that the component must not be used for transfusion if there is abnormal haemolysis or other deterioration;

- that the component must be administered through a 170-200 μm filter.

Storage and stability

As for whole blood.

Removal of buffy coat during component preparation reduces the formation of microaggregates.

Quality assurance

As for whole blood with the exceptions indicated in Table 6.

Table 6: Quality assurance

Parameter to be checked	Quality requirement (specification)	Frequency of control	Control executed by
Volume	250 ± 50 mL	1% of all units	Processing lab
EVF	0.65 to 0.75	4 units per month	QC lab
Haemoglobin	minimum 43 g unit	4 units per month	QC lab
Leucocyte Content/unit*	$<1.2 \times 10^9$	4 units per month	QC lab
Haemolysis at the end of storage	<0.8% of red cell mass	4 units per month	QC lab

*   These requirements shall be deemed to have been met if 75% of the units sampled fall within the values indicated.

Transport

Transport by a non-refrigerated vehicle requires a cooled and insulated container.

Indications for use

Red cells BCR are used for replacement in blood loss and for the therapy of anaemia.

Precautions in use

Compatibility of red cells with the intended recipient must be verified by suitable pre-transfusion testing.

Red cells BCR are not recommended in:

- various types of plasma intolerance;

- exchange transfusions in newborns unless supplementary plasma is added;

- transfusion in premature infants and recipients with a risk of iron overload, unless used within 14 days of donation to reduce frequency of transfusion.

Side-effects

- Circulatory overload.

- Haemolytic transfusion reaction.

- Non-haemolytic transfusion reaction (mainly chills, fever), but less common than after transfusion of red cells.

- Alloimmunisation against HLA and red cell antigens.

- Syphilis can be transmitted when red cells BCR has been stored for less than 96 hours at 4 °C.

- Viral transmission (hepatitis, HIV, etc.) is possible despite careful donor selection and screening procedures.

- Protozoal transmission (e.g. malaria) may occur in rare instances.

- Sepsis due to inadvertent bacterial contamination.

- Biochemical imbalance in massive transfusion, e.g. hyperkalaemia.

- Post-transfusion purpura.

- Transfusion related acute lung injury.

Chapter 7: Red cells, in additive solution (red cells: AS)

Definition

A component derived from whole blood by centrifugation and removal of plasma with subsequent addition to the red cells of an appropriate nutrient solution.

Properties

The EVF of this component will depend on the nature of the additive solution, the method of centrifugation and the amount of remaining plasma. It should not exceed 0.70. Each unit should have a minimum haemoglobin content of 45 g.

The unit contains all of the original unit's red cells. The greater part of its leucocytes (about 2.5 to 3.0×10^9 cells) and a varying content of platelets depending on the method of centrifugation are retained, no effort having been made for removal.

Methods of preparation

The primary anticoagulant solution should be CPD. Most additive solutions contain sodium chloride, adenine, glucose and mannitol dissolved in water. Others contain citrate, mannitol, phosphate and guanosine. The volume may be 80 or 100 mL. Processing should commence as soon as possible after donation (up to a maximum of three days) and be completed in one step.

After centrifugation of the whole blood unit the red cells and plasma are separated. After careful mixing with the additive solution the red cells are stored at 2 °C to 6 °C.

Labelling

The labelling should comply with the relevant national legislation and international agreements. The label on the container states:

-       the name and the volume of the component;

-       the producer's name and address (clear text or code);

-       the donation number;

-       the ABO group;

-       the Rh (D) group, specifying "Rh (D)-positive" if D positive or "Rh (D)-negative" if D negative;

-       the composition and volume of the additive solution;

- the date of collection and expiry date;

- the temperature of storage;

- that the component must not be used for transfusion if there is abnormal haemolysis or other deterioration;

- that the component must be administered through a 170-200 μm filter.

Storage and stability

The same storage conditions are applied as for whole blood and red cells.

Depending on the anticoagulant/additive system the storage may be extended up to the approved limit of the system.

Microaggregates are formed on storage.

Quality assurance

As for whole blood with the exceptions indicated in Table 7.

Table 7: Quality assurance

Parameter to be checked	Quality requirement (specification)	Frequency of control	Control executed by
Volume	to be defined for the system used	1% of all units	Processing lab
EVF	0.50 - 0.70	4 units per month	QC lab
Haemoglobin	minimum 45 g/unit	4 units per month	QC lab
Haemolysis at the end of storage	<0.8% of red cell mass	4 units per month	QC lab

Transport

Transport by a non-refrigerated vehicle requires a cooled and insulated container.

Indications for use

This component is used for replacement in blood loss and for the therapy of anaemia.

Precautions in use

Compatibility of this component with the intended recipient must be verified by suitable pre-transfusion testing.

78

Consideration should be given to the use of a microaggregate filter.

Red cells AS are not recommended in:

-    various types of plasma intolerance (may not concern units with a low plasma content unless IgA incompatibility is present);

-    intolerance due to alloimmunisation against leucocyte antigens;

-    exchange transfusion in newborns unless used within 7 days of donation, with the additive solution replaced by fresh frozen plasma on the day of use;

-    transfusion in premature infants and recipients with a risk of iron overload, unless used within 14 days of donation to reduce frequency of transfusion.

Side-effects

-    Circulatory overload.

-    Haemolytic transfusion reaction.

-    Non-haemolytic transfusion reaction (mainly chills, fever).

-    Alloimmunisation against HLA and red cell antigens.

-    Syphilis can be transmitted when this component has been stored for less than 96 hours at 4 °C.

-    Viral transmission (hepatitis, HIV, etc.) is possible despite careful donor selection and screening procedures.

-    Protozoal transmission (e.g. malaria) may occur in rare instances.

-    Sepsis due to inadvertent bacterial contamination.

-    Biochemical imbalance in massive transfusion, e.g. hyperkalaemia.

-    Post-transfusion purpura.

Chapter 8: Red cells in additive solution, buffy coat removed (red cells: AS-BCR)

Definition

A component derived from whole blood by centrifugation and removal of plasma and buffy coat, and subsequent addition to the red cells of an appropriate nutrient solution.

Properties

The EVF of the component will depend on the nature of the additive solution, the method of centrifugation and the amount of remaining plasma. It should not exceed 0.70. Each unit should have a minimum of 43 g of haemoglobin at the end of processing.

The unit contains all except 20 to 30 mL of the original units' red cells.

The leucocyte content is less than 1.2×10^9 cells per unit and the average platelet content less than 10×10^9 cells per unit.

Methods of preparation

The primary anticoagulant solution should be CPD. Most additive solutions contain sodium chloride, adenine, glucose and mannitol dissolved in water. Others contain citrate, mannitol, phosphate and guanosine. The volume may be 80 or 100 mL. Processing should commence as soon as possible after donation (up to a maximum of 3 days), and be completed in one step.

For the preparation of the component, the plasma and 20 mL to 60 mL of the buffy coat layer are removed from the whole blood after centrifugation.

After careful mixing with the additive solution the red cells are stored at 2 °C to 6 °C.

Labelling

The labelling should comply with the relevant national legislation and international agreements. The label on the container states:

-      the name and the volume of the component;

-      the producer's name and address (clear text or code);

-      the donation number;

-      the ABO group;

- the Rh (D) group, specifying "Rh (D)-positive" if D positive or "Rh (D)-negative" if D negative.

- the composition and volume of the additive solution;

- the date of collection and expiry date;

- the temperature of storage;

- that the component must not be used for transfusion if there is abnormal haemolysis or other deterioration;

- that the component must be administered through a 170-200 μm filter.

Storage and stability

The same storage conditions are applied as for whole blood and red cells.

Depending on the anticoagulant/additive system the storage may be extended to the approved limit of the system.

Removal of buffy coat during component preparation reduces the formation of microaggregates.

Quality assurance

As for whole blood, with the exceptions indicated in Table 8.

Table 8: Quality assurance

Parameter to be checked	Quality requirement	Frequency of control	Control executed by
Volume	to be defined for the system used	1% of all units	Processing lab
EVF	0.50 - 0.70	4 units per month	QC lab
Haemoglobin	minimum 43 g/unit	4 units per month	QC lab
Leucocyte Content/unit *	$<1.2 \times 10^9$	4 units per month	QC lab
Haemolysis at the end of storage	<0.8% of red cell mass	4 units per month	QC lab

* These requirements shall be deemed to have been met if 75% of the units sampled fall within the values indicated.

Transport

Transport by a non-refrigerated vehicle requires a cooled and insulated container.

Indications for use

Red cells AS-BCR are used for replacement in blood loss and for the therapy of anaemia.

Precautions in use

Compatibility of this component with the intended recipient must be verified by suitable pre-transfusion testing.

Red cells AS-BCR are not recommended in:

- various types of plasma intolerance (may not apply to units with a low plasma content);

- exchange transfusions in newborns unless used within 7 days of donation, with the additive solution replaced by fresh frozen plasma on the day of use;

- transfusion in premature infants and recipients with a risk of iron overload, unless used within 14 days of donation to reduce frequency of transfusion.

Side-effects

- Circulatory overload.

- Haemolytic transfusion reaction.

- Non-haemolytic transfusion reaction (mainly chills, fever) but are less common than after transfusion of red cells AS.

- Alloimmunisation against HLA and red cell antigens.

- Syphilis can be transmitted when this component has been stored for less than 96 hours at 4 °C.

- Viral transmission (hepatitis, HIV, etc.) is possible despite careful donor selection and screening procedures.

- Protozoal transmission (e.g. malaria) may occur in rare instances.

- Sepsis due to inadvertent bacterial contamination.

- Biochemical imbalance in massive transfusion, e.g. hyperkalaemia.

- Post-transfusion purpura.

Chapter 9: Washed red cells

Definition

A component derived from whole blood by centrifugation and removal of plasma, with subsequent washing of the red cells in an isotonic solution.

Properties

This component is a red cell suspension from which most of the plasma, leucocytes and platelets have been removed. The amount of residual plasma will depend upon the washing protocol. The EVF can be varied according to clinical need. Each unit should have a minimum of 40 g of haemoglobin at the end of processing.

Methods of preparation

After centrifugation and maximal removal of plasma and buffy coat, the red cells are processed by sequential addition of cold (4 °C) isotonic saline and refrigerated centrifugation. A functionally closed system can be prepared by using a sterile connecting device.

Labelling

The labelling should comply with the relevant national legislation and international agreements. The label on the container states:

- time of preparation and expiry;

- the name and the volume of the component;

- the producer's name and address (clear text or code);

- the donation number;

- the ABO group;

- the Rh (D) group, specifying "Rh (D)-positive" if D positive or "Rh (D)-negative" if D negative.

- the composition and volume of the suspending solution;

- the temperature of storage;

- that the component must not be used for transfusion if there is abnormal haemolysis or other deterioration;

- that the component must be administered through a 170-200 μm filter.

Storage and stability

The component should be stored at 2 °C to 6 °C. The storage time should be as short as possible after washing and certainly not longer than 24 hours provided low temperature preparation has been observed. Storage should be no longer than 6 hours if preparation has been at room temperature.

Quality assurance

As for whole blood, with the exceptions indicated in Table 9.

Table 9: Quality assurance

Parameter to be checked	Quality requirement	Frequency of control	Control executed by
Volume	280 + 60 mL	all units	Processing lab
EVF	0.65 to 0.75	all units	QC lab
Haemoglobin	minimum 40 g/unit	all units	QC lab
Haemolysis at end of storage	<0.8% of red cell mass	all units	QC lab
Protein content	<0.5 g/unit*	all units	QC lab

*   this level of total protein should ensure an IgA content of less than 0.2 mg/unit.

Transport

Transport is limited by the short storage time. Storage conditions should be maintained during transportation. Attention to strict control of temperature and time is required.

Indications for use

Washed red cells are only indicated for red cell substitution or replacement in patients with plasma protein antibodies, especially anti-IgA, and in patients who have shown severe allergic reactions in association with transfusion of blood products.

Precautions in use

Compatibility of the washed red cell suspension with the intended recipient must be verified by a suitable pretransfusion testing.

Side-effects

- Circulatory overload.

- Haemolytic transfusion reaction.

- Alloimmunisation against HLA and red cell antigens.

- Syphilis can be transmitted if the component is prepared from a blood unit which has been stored for less than 96 hours at 2 °C to 6 °C.

- Viral transmission (hepatitis, HIV, etc.) is possible despite careful donor selection and screening procedures.

- Protozoal transmission (e.g. malaria) may occur in rare instances.

- Sepsis due to inadvertent bacterial contamination.

- Post-transfusion purpura.

Chapter 10: Red cells, leucocyte-depleted

Definition

A component obtained by removing the majority of leucocytes from a red cell preparation.

Properties

The leucocyte count must be less than 1×10^6 per unit. Mean counts as low as 0.05×10^6 are achievable. Each unit should have a minimum haemoglobin content of 40 g.

Methods of preparation

Various techniques are used to produce this preparation including buffy coat depletion and filtration. The best results are currently achieved using a combination of both these methods.

A fully validated procedure must be established to determine optimum conditions for use of the leucocyte depletion method.

Pre-storage filtration is recommended, preferably within 48 hours after donation.

Labelling

The labelling should comply with the relevant national legislation and international agreements. The label on the container states:

-       the name and the volume of the component;

-       the producer's name and address (clear text or code);

-       the donation number;

-       the ABO group;

-       the Rh (D) group, specifying "Rh (D)-positive" if D positive or "Rh (D)-negative" if D negative;

-       the composition and volume of the anticoagulant solution;

-       the date of collection and expiry date;

-       the temperature of storage;

- that the component must not be used for transfusion if there is abnormal haemolysis or other deterioration;

- that the component must be administered through a 170-200 µm filter.

Storage and stability

The same storage conditions are applied as for whole blood and red cells.

Removal of leucocytes before storage reduces the formation of microaggregates.

Red cells leucocyte-depleted, if filtered or prepared by other methods under which the system has been opened, have a storage life limited to 24 hours at 2 °C to 6 °C.

Quality assurance

As for whole blood, with the exceptions indicated in Table 10.

Table 10: Quality assurance

Parameter to be checked	Quality requirement	Frequency of control	Control executed by
Residual white cells *	$<1 \times 10^6$ per unit by count	4 units per month or 1% of units, whichever is higher	QC lab
Haemoglobin	min 40 g/unit	4 units per month or 1%, whichever is higher	QC lab

* These requirements shall be deemed to have been met if 90% of the units sampled fall within the values indicated.

Transport

Similar principles as for whole blood and other red cell components will apply. Attention to strict control of temperature and time is required where an open system of preparation has been used.

Indications for use

The same indications as for red cells apply. This component is indicated for patients with known or suspected leucocyte antibodies or whose transfusion requirement is likely to be ongoing to prevent alloimmunisation to leucocyte antibodies.

This component is an acceptable alternative to CMV negative blood for prevention of CMV transmission.

Precautions in use

Compatibility of this component with the intended recipient must be verified by suitable pre-transfusion testing.

This component is expected to have very low HLA immunogenicity and reduced risk of CMV transmission and not to cause reactions in individuals immunised against leucocytes, provided other components used are also leucocyte depleted.

Red cells leucocyte depleted are not recommended in:

- various types of plasma intolerance (may not apply to units with a low plasma content);

- exchange transfusion in newborns unless used within 5 days of donation;

- transfusion in premature infants and recipients with a risk of iron overload, unless used within 14 days of donation to reduce frequency of transfusion.

Side-effects

- Circulatory overload.

- Haemolytic transfusion reaction.

- Non-haemolytic transfusion reaction (mainly chills, fever), less common than after transfusion of whole blood or other red cell components.

- Alloimmunisation against HLA (rarely) and red cell antigens.

- Syphilis can be transmitted when this product has been stored for less than 96 hours at 4 °C.

- Viral transmission (hepatitis, HIV, etc.) is possible despite careful donor selection and screening procedures.

- Protozoal transmission (e.g. malaria) may occur in rare instances.

- Sepsis due to inadvertent bacterial contamination.

- Biochemical imbalance in massive transfusion, e.g. hyperkalaemia.

- Post-transfusion purpura.

- Transfusion related acute lung injury.

Chapter 11: Cryopreserved red cells

Definition

A component derived from whole blood, in which red cells are frozen, preferably within 7 days of collection, using a cryoprotectant, and stored at -80 °C or below. Before use the cells are thawed, washed and suspended in isotonic sodium chloride solution.

Properties

A reconstituted unit of cryopreserved red cells is practically free of protein, granulocytes and platelets. Each reconstituted unit should have a minimum haemoglobin content of 36 g.

Methods of preparation

Two principles are in general use for preparation of cryopreserved red cells. One is a high glycerol (40% w/v), the other a low glycerol (17% w/v) technique. Both methods require a washing/deglycerolisation procedure.

Labelling

The labelling should comply with the relevant national legislation and international agreements. The label on the container states:

- the date and time of preparation and expiry;

- the name and the volume of the component;

- the producer's name and address (clear text or code);

- the donation number;

- the ABO group;

- the Rh (D) group, specifying "Rh (D)-positive" if D positive or "Rh (D)-negative" if D negative;

- the composition and volume of the suspending solution;

- the temperature of storage;

- that the component must not be used for transfusion if there is abnormal haemolysis or other deterioration;

- that the component must be administered through a 170-200 μm filter.

Extra caution should be applied in identification of frozen bag units.

Storage and stability

Red cells in frozen state

These should be constantly maintained at:

-   minus 60 °C to minus 80 °C if stored in an electrical freezer when a high glycerol method is used;

-   minus 140 °C to minus 150 °C if stored in vapour phase liquid nitrogen, when a low glycerol method is used.

The storage may be extended to at least ten years if the correct storage temperature can be guaranteed.

Thawed reconstituted red cells

The product should be stored at 2 °C to 6 °C. The storage time should be as short as possible after washing and never exceed 24 hours when an open system has been used.

Quality assurance

As for whole blood, with the exceptions indicated in Table 11.

Table 11: Quality assurance

Parameter to be checked	Quality requirement (specification)	Frequency of control	Control executed by
Volume	> 185 ml	all units	Processing lab
Hb (supernatant) *	< 0.2 g/unit	all units	QC lab
EVF	0.65 - 0.75	all units	QC lab
Haemoglobin	> 36 g/unit	all units	QC lab
Osmolarity	< 340 mOsm/1	5% of units	Processing lab
Leucocyte **	$< 0.1 \times 10^9$	1% of units	QC lab
Sterility	Sterile	all units	QC lab

*   Final suspending solution.
** These requirements shall have been deemed to have been met if 75% of the units sampled fall within the values indicated.

Excess haemolysis should not be observed in the washing solution at the end of the washing procedure.

Transport

If transport in the frozen state is unavoidable, storage conditions should be maintained.

Transport of thawed reconstituted red cells is limited by the short storage time. Storage conditions should be maintained during transport.

Indications for use

Cryopreserved red cells are indicated for red cell substitution or replacement. This component should only be used in special situations:

- transfusion of red cells to patients with rare blood types/multiple alloantibodies;

- may also be used when CMV negative red cell preparations or leukocyte depleted red cells are indicated but not available;

- red cells cryopreserved for at least six months are recommended for immunisation purposes, to allow retesting of donors;

- could be considered in some cases for autologous transfusion.

Precautions in use

Compatibility of the washed red cell suspension with the intended recipient must be verified by a suitable pretransfusion testing.

When processing in an open system, the risk of bacterial contamination is increased and therefore extra vigilance is required during transfusion.

Side-effects

- Circulatory overload.

- Protozoal transmission (e.g. malaria) may occur in rare instances.

- Viral transmission (hepatitis, HIV, etc), is possible despite careful donor selection and screening procedures.

- Alloimmunisation against red cell antigens.

- Sepsis due to inadvertent bacterial contamination.

Chapter 12: Platelets: recovered

Definition

A component derived from fresh whole blood which contains the majority of the original platelet content in a therapeutically effective form.

Properties

Depending on the method of preparation, the platelet content per single unit equivalent will vary from 45 to 85 $\times$ 10^9 (on average 70 $\times$ 10^9) in 50 to 60 mL suspension medium. Similarly, leucocyte content will vary from 0.05 to 1 $\times$ 10^9 and red cells from 0.2 to 1 $\times$ 10^9 per single unit equivalent, unless further measures are taken to reduce these numbers.

The amount of platelets in a "standard unit" of recovered platelets is equivalent to the amount obtained from 4 to 6 units of whole blood.

Methods of preparation

1.   Preparation of platelet-rich plasma (PRP)

Principle: a unit of fresh blood is centrifuged so that an optimal number of platelets remain in plasma and the number of leucocytes and red cells are reduced to a defined level. The key points of the method are:

   a.   effectiveness of centrifugation defined as g $\times$ min;

   b.   temperature of the blood during centrifugation must be standardised;

   c.   disturbance of the component layers achieved by centrifugation must be avoided;

   d.   in removing the supernatant plasma the flow should not be too rapid and the separation must be stopped at the level of 8 to 10 mm above the surface of the red cell layer.

2.   Preparation of platelets from platelet-rich plasma

Principle: platelets in PRP are sedimented by heavy centrifugation; the supernatant platelet-poor plasma is removed leaving 50-70 mL of it with the platelets; finally the platelets are allowed to disaggregate and are then resuspended.

3. *Preparation of platelets from buffy coat*

Principle: a fresh blood unit is centrifuged so that blood platelets are primarily sedimented to the buffy coat layer together with leucocytes. The buffy coat is separated and further processed to obtain a platelet concentrate. Either single buffy coats or pooled (4 to 6) buffycoats are diluted with plasma or an appropriate nutrient solution. After careful mixing, the buffy coat or buffy coat pool is centrifuged so that platelets remain in the supernatant but red cells and leucocytes are effectively sedimented to the bottom of the bag. The key points of the method are similar to those mentioned for PRP.

Leucocyte-depleted platelets can be prepared by filtration , pre-storage leucocyte depletion is recommended (preferably within 6 hours after recovery).

A fully validated procedure must be established to determine optimum conditions for the leucocyte depletion method used.

Where necessary, volume-reduced or washed platelets can be prepared.

Labelling

The labelling should comply with the relevant national legislation and international agreements. The label on the container states:

- the name of the component;

- the producer's name and address (clear text or code);

- the donation number (if platelets are pooled a system of labelling must be employed that allows identification of the original donations);

- date of collection and expiry;

- recommended storage temperature;

- the ABO group;

- the Rh (D) group specifying "Rh (D)-positive" if D positive or "Rh (D)-negative" if D negative;

- volume of content and average number of platelets;

- whether or not leucocyte depleted;

- nature of anticoagulant and diluting solution;

- that the component must be administered throughout a 170-200 μm filter.

Storage and stability

Platelets must be stored under conditions which guarantee that their viability and haemostatic activities are optimally preserved.

Plastic bags intended for platelet storage must be sufficiently permeable to gases to guarantee availability of oxygen to platelets. The amount of oxygen required is dependent on the concentration of platelets and leucocytes in the product. The volume of the dilution solution used must be large enough to guarantee that the concentration of platelets is <1.5 X 10^9/mL and the pH of the platelet product stays continuously between 6.5 and 7.4 under the storage conditions used.

Agitation of platelets during storage must be efficient enough to guarantee availability of oxygen but be as gentle as possible. Storage temperature should be 22 °C (+/-2 °C).

Viability of platelets is preserved up to seven days under optimal conditions. However, more than five days' storage of platelets is not at present recommended.

Quality assurance

Demonstration of the swirling phenomenon, based on light scattering by platelets of normal morphology in movement, may be carried out either as a separate quality control procedure or as a routine part of the issue and transfusion of this component.

Quality control requirements as for whole blood with the additions shown in Table 12.

Table 12

Parameter to be checked	Quality requirement (specification)	Frequency of control	Control executed by
HLA or HPA (when required)	Typing	as required	HLA lab
Volume	> 50 mL	all units	processing lab
Platelet Count*	> 60 × 10^9/single unit equivalent	5% of issued units with a minimum of 4 units/month	QC lab
Residual leucocytes* before leucocyte depletion			
a. prepared from PRP	< 0.2 × 10^9/single unit equivalent	1% of units with a minimum of 4 units/month	QC lab
b. prepared from buffy coat	< 0.05 × 10^9/single unit equivalent		
Residual leucocytes** after leucocytes depletion	< 0.2 × 10^6/single unit equivalent	5% of units ≥ 10/month	QC lab
pH measured (+22 °C/closed system) at the end of the recommended shelf life	6.5 to 7.4	1% of all units with a minimum of 4 units/month	QC lab

* These requirements shall be deemed to have been met if 75% of the units sampled fall within the values indicated.

** These requirements shall be deemed to have been met if 90% of the units sampled fall within the values indicated.

Transport

Containers for transporting platelets should be kept open at room temperature for 30 minutes before use. During transportation the temperature of platelet components must be kept as close as possible to recommended storage temperature and, on receipt, unless intended for immediate therapeutic use, they should be transferred to storage under recommended conditions. It is recommended that they be further agitated prior to use.

Indications for use

The decision to transfuse platelets should not be based on low platelet count alone. A mandatory indication may be considered to be the presence of severe thrombocytopenia, with clinically significant haemorrhage attributable to the platelet deficit. All other indications for platelet transfusion are more or less relative and dependent on the clinical condition of the patient.

Precautions in use

Upon pre-storage pooling (either buffy coats or platelet suspensions) platelets may be stored for up to 5 days following donation. If the pooling of platelets is performed after storage, platelets should be transfused as soon as possible but no later than 6 hours after pooling.

Rh (D) negative female recipients of child bearing age or younger should preferably not be transfused with platelets from Rh (D) positive donors. If platelets from Rh (D) positive donors must be used in these circumstances the prevention of Rh (D) immunisation by the use of Rh-immune globulin should be considered.

Side-effects

-   Non-haemolytic transfusion reactions may occur (mainly chills, fever and urticaria). The incidence will be reduced by the use of leucocyte depleted platelets.

-   Alloimmunisation, especially to the HLA and HPA antigens, may occur. When leucocyte-depleted platelets are used, the risk of HLA alloimmunisation is reduced, provided that other transfused components are also leucocyte depleted.

-   Syphilis can be transmitted.

-   Viral transmission (hepatitis, HIV, etc.) is possible despite careful donor selection and laboratory screening procedures. However, risks of CMV transmission can be reduced by leucocyte depletion.

-   Protozoal transmission (e.g. malaria) may occur in rare instances.

-   Sepsis due to inadvertent bacterial contamination.

- Post-transfusion purpura may occur.

- Transfusion related acute lung injury when platelets are suspended in plasma.

Chapter 13: Platelets: apheresis

Definition

A component obtained by platelet apheresis of a single donor using automated cell separation equipment.

Properties

Depending on the method of preparation and the machine used, the platelet yield per procedure will vary from 200 to 800×10^9. Similarly, leucocyte and red cell contamination of the product may vary with the procedure and type of machine used. The method provides the ability to collect platelets from selected donors, to reduce risk of HLA alloimmunisation and for effective treatment of patients already alloimmunised. By reducing the number of donor exposures, the risk of viral transmission may also be reduced.

A standard unit should be the equivalent of 5 single donors units of recovered platelets.

Methods of preparation

In platelet apheresis, whole blood is removed from the donor, platelets are harvested from it by the apheresis machine and the remaining blood components are returned to the donor. To reduce the number of contaminating leucocytes an additional centrifugation or filtration step may be included in the process.

With apheresis, the equivalent of platelets obtained from 3 to 13 whole blood units can be collected from a single procedure and can be divided into several standard units for transfusion.

Labelling

The labelling should comply with the relevant national legislation and international agreements. The label on the container states:

- the name of the component;

- the producer's name and address (clear text or code);

- the donation number;

- date of collection and expiry;

- recommended storage temperature;

- the ABO group;

- the Rh (D) group specifying "Rh (D)-positive" if D positive or "Rh (D)-negative" if D negative;

- volume of content and average number of platelets except that the actual number should be indicated if the unit does not meet the recommended standard;

- that the component must be administered through a 170-200 μm filter if pooling or leucocyte depletion has been carried out.

Storage and stability

Platelets must be stored under conditions which guarantee that their viability and haemostatic activities are optimally preserved.

Platelet components to be stored more than 24 hours must be collected and prepared in a functionally closed system.

Plastic bags intended for platelet storage must be sufficiently permeable to gases to guarantee availability of oxygen to platelets. The amount of oxygen required is dependent on the concentration of platelets and leucocytes in the product. Volume of plasma must be large enough (more than $1 \text{ mL}/1.5 \times 10^9$ platelets) to guarantee that the pH of the platelet suspension stays continuously between 6.5 and 7.4 under the storage conditions used.

Agitation of platelets during storage must be efficient enough to guarantee availability of oxygen but be as gentle as possible.

Temperature: 22 °C ± 2 °C.

Viability of platelets is preserved up to seven days under optimal conditions. However, storage of platelets for more than five days is not presently recommended.

Quality assurance

Demonstration of the swirling phenomenon, based on light scattering by platelets of normal morphology in movement, may be carried out either as a separate quality control procedure or as a routine part of the issue and transfusion of these products.

Quality control requirements as for whole blood with the additions shown in Table 13(a).

Table 13(a): Quality assurance

Parameter to be checked	Quality requirement	Frequency of control	Control executed by
ABO, Rh (D)	grouping	all units	grouping lab
HLA or HPA (when required)	typing	as required	HLA lab
HIV-Abs	negative by approved screening test	all units	screening lab
HBsAg	negative by approved screening test	all units	screening lab
ALT (when required)	not elevated (as specified by national authorities)	all units	screening lab
HBc-Ab (when required)	negative by approved screening test	all units	screening lab
Syphilis (when required)	negative by screening test	all units	screening lab
CMV-Ab (when required)	negative by screening test	as required	screening lab
HCV-Ab	negative by approved screening test	all units	screening lab
HTLV-Abs (when required)	negative by screening test	all units	screening lab

Table 13(b)

Parameter to be checked	Quality requirement	Frequency of control	Control executed by
Volume	> 40 mL per 60.10^9 platelets	all units	processing lab
Platelet count*	> 300 × 10^9/unit	5% of all units with a minimum of 4 units/month	QC lab
Residual leucocytes*		5% of all units with a minimum of 4 units/month	QC lab
- before leucocyte depletion*	< 1.0 × 10^9 per standard unit		
- after leucocyte depletion**	< 1.0 × 10^6 per standard unit		
pH measured end of recommended shelf life	6.5 to 7.4 (+22 °C/closed system)	1% of all units with a minimum of 4 units/month	QC lab

* The requirements shall be deemed to have been met if 75% of the units sampled fall within the values indicated. Residual leucocyte values much lower than these are obtainable with some apheresis machines.

** The requirements shall be deemed to have been met if 90% of the units sampled fall within the values indicated. Residual leucocyte values much lower than these are obtainable with some apheresis machines.

Transport

Containers for transporting platelets should be kept open at room temperature for 30 minutes before use. During transportation the temperature of platelet components must be kept as close as possible to recommended storage temperature and, on receipt, unless intended for immediate therapeutic use, they should be transferred to storage under recommended conditions. It is recommended that they be further agitated prior to use.

Indications for use

The decision to transfuse platelets should not be based on low platelet count alone. A mandatory indication may be considered to be the presence of severe thrombocytopenia, with clinically significant haemorrhage attributable to the platelet deficit. All other indications for platelet transfusion are more or less relative and dependent on the clinical condition of the patient. HLA and/or HPA compatible platelets may be useful in the treatment of immunised patients. It is recommended that these should not be obtained by apheresis of relatives of the patient or other HLA match individual who are potential haematopoietic progenitor stem cell donors.

Precautions in use

Rh negative female recipients of child-bearing age or younger should not be transfused with platelets from Rh-positive donors. If platelets from Rh (D)-positive donors must be used in these circumstances the prevention of Rh (D) immunisation by the use of Rh-immune globulin should be considered.

The responsible physician should be informed if a unit of apheresis platelets which does not meet the recommended standards for platelets content must be issued for therapeutic use.

Platelets compatibility testing may be useful in the selection of platelets for transfusion to an immunised patient.

Side-effects

- Non-haemolytic transfusion reactions may occur (mainly chills, fever and urticaria). The incidence will be reduced by the use of leucocyte depleted platelets.

- Alloimmunisation especially to the HLA and HPA series of antigens may occur. When leucocyte-depleted platelets are used, the risk of HLA alloimmunisation is reduced provided other components used are also leucocyte depleted.

- Syphilis can be transmitted.

- Viral transmission (hepatitis, HIV, etc.) is possible despite careful donor selection and laboratory screening procedures.

- Protozoal transmission (e.g. malaria) may occur in rare instances.

- Sepsis due to inadvertent bacterial contamination.

- Post-transfusion purpura may occur.

- Transfusion related acute lung injury.

Chapter 14: Fresh frozen plasma

Definition

A component for transfusion prepared either from whole blood or from plasma collected by apheresis, frozen within a period and to a temperature that will adequately maintain the labile coagulation factors in a functional state.

Properties

This preparation contains normal plasma levels of stable coagulation factors, albumin and immunoglobulins. It contains a minimum of 70% of the original Factor VIIIc and at least similar quantities of the other labile coagulation factors and naturally occurring inhibitors. If fresh frozen plasma is to be used as source material for the preparation of fractionated products, reference should be made to the European Pharmacopoeia monograph on plasma for fractionation.

Methods of preparation

a. Whole blood

Plasma is separated from whole blood collected using a blood bag with integral transfer packs, employing heavy spin centrifugation, preferably within 6 hours and not more than 18 hours after collection. Plasma may also be separated from platelet rich plasma. Freezing should take place in a system that will allow complete freezing within one hour to a temperature below -30 °C. If plasma is to be prepared from a single pack whole blood donation, adequate sterility precautions must be adopted.

Where Health Authorities allow, plasma may also be separated from whole blood, which immediately after donation has been rapidly cooled by special device between +20 °C and +22 °C and held at that temperature for up to 24 hours, depending on the nature of the anticoagulant used.

b. By apheresis

Plasma may be collected by manual or automated apheresis. The freezing process should commence within one hour of completion of the procedure.

c. Viral inactivation

Viral inactivation and/or quarantine of these components are a requirement in some countries.

Labelling

The labelling should comply with the relevant national legislation and international agreements. The label in the container states:

- name of component;

- nature of component, i.e. from a whole blood donation or by apheresis. The volume should be stated and the nature of the anticoagulant used;

- donation number;

- the ABO group;

- the Rh (D) group specifying "Rh (D)-positive" if D positive or "Rh (D)-negative" if D negative;

- the producer's name and address (clear text or code);

- whether quarantine or viral inactivated.

The following additional information may be placed on the pack or alternatively on a container surrounding the pack (i.e plasma container carton):

- date of preparation;

- storage temperature and expiry date;

- instructions for restorage, thawing and administration including the use of a standard filter.

Storage and stability

The stability on storage is dependent on the storage temperature available. Optimal storage temperature is at -30 °C or lower and the following are the permitted storage times and temperatures:

24 months at -40 °C or below
12 months at -30 °C to -40 °C
6 months at -25 °C to -30 °C
3 months at -18 °C to -25 °C

Quality assurance

Table 14(a)

Parameter to be checked	Quality requirement (specification)	Frequency of control	Control executed by
ABO, Rh (D)*	grouping	all units	grouping lab
HIV-Abs*	negative by approved screening test	all units	screening lab
HBsAg*	negative by approved screening test	all units	screening lab
ALT* (when required)	not elevated (as specified by national authorities)	all units	screening lab
HCV-Ab*	negative by approved screening test	all units	screening lab
HBc-Abs* (when required)	negative by approved screening test	all units	screening lab
Syphilis* (when required)	negative by screening test	all units	screening lab
HTLV-Abs* (when required)	negative by screening test	all units	screening lab

Table 14(b)

Parameter to be checked	Quality requirement (specification)	Frequency of control	Control executed by
Volume	stated volume ± 10%	all units	processing lab
Factor VIIIc	> 0.7 i.u./mL	every two months. a) pool of 6 units of mixed blood groups during first month of storage. b) pool of 6 units of mixed blood groups during last month of storage	QC lab
Residual cells**	red cells: < 6.0 × 10⁹/1 leucocytes:< 0.1 × 10⁹/1 platelets: < 50 × 10⁹/1	1% of all units with a minimum of 4 units/month	QC lab
Leakage	no leakage at any part of container e.g. visual inspection after pressure in a plasma extractor, before freezing and after thawing	all units	processing and receiving laboratory
Visual changes	no abnormal colour or visible clots	all units	"

*   Unless performed on whole blood used as the source.
**   Cell counting performed before freezing. Low levels can be achieved if specific cellular depletions are included in the protocol.

Note   If fresh frozen plasma is regularly used as a source of a component other than Factor VIIIc, appropriate estimations should be performed on representative sample units to ensure continuing efficiency of the preparative procedure.

Transport

Storage temperature should be maintained during transport. The receiving hospital should ensure that packs have remained frozen during transit. Unless for immediate use, the packs should be transferred at once to storage at the recommended temperature.

Indications for use

Fresh frozen plasma may be used in coagulation disorders, particularly in those clinical situations in which a multiple coagulation deficit exists and only where no suitable viral inactivated alternative is available.

Fresh frozen plasma may be used in the treatment of thrombic thrombocytopenic purpura (TTP).

Its major use is as source material for plasma fractionation.

Precautions in use

Fresh frozen plasma should not be used simply to correct a volume deficit in the absence of a coagulation deficit nor as a source of immunoglobulins.

Fresh frozen plasma should not be used where a suitable viral inactivated alternative product is available.

Fresh frozen plasma should not be used in a patient with intolerance to plasma proteins.

Blood group-compatible plasma should be used.

The product should be used immediately following thawing. It should not be refrozen.

Before use the product should be thawed in a properly controlled environment and the integrity of the pack should be verified to exclude any defects or leakages. No insoluble cryoprecipitate should be visible on completion of the thaw procedure.

Side-effects

-        Citrate toxicity can occur when large volumes are rapidly transfused;

-        Non-haemolytic transfusion reactions (mainly chills, fever and urticaria);

-        Viral transmission (hepatitis, HIV, etc,) is possible despite careful donor selection and screening procedures;

-        Sepsis due to inadvertent bacterial contamination;

-        Transfusion related acute lung injury.

Chapter 15: Cryoprecipitate

Definition

A component containing the cryoglobulin fraction of plasma obtained by further processing of fresh frozen plasma prepared from hard-spun cell free plasma and concentrated to a final volume of 10 to 20 mL.

Properties

Contains a major portion of the Factor VIII, von Willebrand factor, fibrinogen, Factor XIII and fibronectin present in freshly drawn and separated plasma.

Methods of preparation

The frozen plasma pack, still attached to other integral (or connected by a sterile docking device) satellite pack(s) and/or the primary blood pack, is allowed to thaw, either overnight at 2 °C to 6 °C or by the rapid-thaw syphon technique.

Following slow-thaw at 2 °C to 6 °C, the pack system is recentrifuged using heavy spin at the same temperature, the supernatant cryo-poor plasma then being expressed on to the donor red cells or into a separate satellite pack. By either thawing and separation technique, 7 to 10 mL supernatant plasma is left with the cryoprecipitate. The components prepared are then separated from each other using a secure, approved method for dividing the transfer tubing refrozen to the appropriate core temperature and held under appropriate storage conditions.

Alternatively, plasma obtained by apheresis may be used as the starting material, the final component being prepared by the same freezing/thawing/refreezing technique.

Labelling

The labelling should comply with the relevant national legislation and international agreements. The label on the container states:

- the name of the component;

- the nature of the component, i.e. from a whole blood donation or by apheresis;

- the donation number;

- the ABO group;

- the Rh (D) group specifying "Rh (D)-positive" if D positive or "Rh (D)-negative" if D negative;

- the producer's name and address (clear text or code).

The following additional information may be placed on the pack or alternatively on a container surrounding the pack:

- date of preparation;

- storage temperature and expiry date;

- instructions on storage, thawing and administration including the use of a standard filter.

Storage and stability

The stability on storage is dependent on the storage temperature available. Optimal storage temperature is -30 °C and the following are permitted storage times and temperatures:

24 months at -40 °C or below
12 months at -30 °C to -40 °C
6 months at -25 °C to -30 °C
3 months at -18 °C to -25 °C

Quality assurance

As indicated in Table 14a with the following additions:

Table 15

Parameter to be checked	Quality requirement	Frequency of control	Control executed by
Estimated volume	10 to 20 mL	all units	processing lab
Factor VIIIc	> 70 i.u/unit	every two months: a. pool of 6 units of mixed blood groups during first month of storage b. pool of 6 units of mixed blood groups during last month of storage	QC lab
Fibrinogen	> 140 mg per unit	1% of all units	QC lab

Note If cryoprecipitate is regularly used as a source of a component other than Factor VIIIc, appropriate estimations should be performed on representative sample units to ensure continuing efficiency of the preparative procedure.

Transport

Storage temperature should be maintained during transport. The receiving hospital should ensure that packs have remained frozen during transit. Unless for immediate use, the packs should be transferred at once to storage at the recommended temperature.

Indications for use

Uses include:

a. Factor VIII deficiency states (haemophilia A, Von Willebrand disease where a suitable viral inactivated product is not available);

b. disseminated intravascular coagulation;

c. fibrinogen defects (quantitative and qualitative);

d. as a substrate for fibrin sealant.

Precautions in use

The pack of cryoprecipitate should be thawed in a properly controlled environment at 37 °C immediately after removal from storage and immediately before use. Dissolving of the precipitate should be encouraged by careful manipulation during the thawing procedure.

At low temperatures the plastic container may fracture and during thawing the pack should be carefully inspected for leaks, and discarded if any are found.

The pack should not be re-frozen.

In rare instances, haemolysis of recipient red blood cells due to high titre alloagglutinins in the donor have been recorded.

Side-effects

-   Non-haemolytic transfusion reactions (mainly chills, fever and urticaria).

-   Possibility of development of inhibitors to Factor VIII in the haemophiliac.

-   Viral transmission (hepatitis, HIV, etc.) is possible despite careful donor selection and screening procedures.

-   Sepsis due to inadvertent bacterial contamination.

Small pool preparations

In some situations, it may be desirable to pool up to 10 single-donor cryoprecipitate units. If this is carried out by an open technique, the pool should be used within 1 hour, and not re-frozen for further storage. Appropriate labelling of the pool must ensure that its individual constituents can be traced without difficulty.

Chapter 16: Cryoprecipitate-depleted plasma

Definition

A component prepared from plasma by the removal of cryoprecipitate.

Properties

Its content of albumin, immunoglobulins and coagulation factors is the same as that of fresh frozen plasma, except that the levels of the labile Factors V and VIII are markedly reduced. The fibrinogen concentration is also reduced in comparison to fresh frozen plasma.

Method of preparation

Cryoprecipitate-depleted plasma is the by-product of the preparation of cryoprecipitate from fresh frozen plasma.

Labelling

The labelling should comply with the relevant national legislation and international agreements. The label on the container states:

–   the name of the component;

–   the nature of component, i.e. from a whole blood donation or by apheresis and the nature of the anticoagulant used;

–   the donation number;

–   the ABO group;

–   the Rh (D) group specifying "Rh (D)-positive" if D positive or "Rh (D)-negative" if D negative;

–   the producer's name and address (clear text or code);

–   volume.

The following additional information may be placed on the pack or alternatively on a container surrounding the pack (i.e. plasma container carton):

–   date of preparation;

–   storage temperature and expiry date;

119

–   instructions for storage, thawing and administration including the use of a standard filter.

Storage and stability

Cryoprecipitate-depleted plasma may be stored at 2 °C to 6 °C for a maximum of 14 days when prepared in a closed system, or may be kept frozen for up to 12 months at -20 °C to -30 °C or up to 24 months below -30 °C.

Quality assurance

As indicated in Table 14a with the following additions:

Table 16

Parameter to be checked	Quality requirement	Frequency of control	Control executed by
Volume	stated volume ± 10%	all units	processing lab

Transport

Storage temperature should be maintained during transport. The receiving hospital should ensure that frozen packs have remained frozen during transit. Unless for immediate use, the packs should be transferred at once to storage at the recommended temperature.

Indications for use

Cryoprecipitate-depleted plasma is indicated in TTP only.

Precautions in use

The routine use of this material is not encouraged because of the risk of viral transmission, and the general availability of safer alternatives.

This product should not be used in a patient with intolerance to plasma protein. Blood group compatible plasma should be used. The product should be used immediately following thawing, it should not be refrozen.

If cryoprecipitate-depleted plasma has been frozen after production, flocculation can occur upon re-thawing. Before freezing and after thawing, the pack should be carefully inspected for leaks.

Side-effects

–   Non-haemolytic transfusion reaction (mainly chills, fever and urticaria).

–   Citrate toxicity can occur when large volumes are rapidly transfused.

120

-   Viral transmission (hepatitis, HIV, etc.) is possible despite careful donor selection and screening procedures.

-   Sepsis due to inadvertent bacterial contamination.

-   Transfusion related acute lung injury.

Chapter 17: Cryopreserved platelets: apheresis

Definition

A component prepared by the freezing of platelets within 24 hours of collection, using a cryoprotectant, storing them at -80 °C or below.

Properties

A reconstituted unit of cryopreserved platelets is practically free of red cells and granulocytes. The method provides the ability to store platelets from selected donors or for autologous use.

Method of preparation

Two methods are in general use for preparation of cryopreserved platelets. One is a DMSO (6% w/v), the other a very low glycerol (5% w/v), technique.

Before use the platelets are thawed and washed (or suspended) in autologous platelet poor plasma or in isotonic sodium chloride solution.

Labelling

1. *Platelets in the frozen state*

Extra caution should be applied in identification of the bags.

2. *Thawed unit*

The labelling should comply with the relevant national legislation and international agreements. The label of the container states:

− the name of the component;

− the producer's name and address (clear text or code);

− the donation number;

− date of preparation and expiry;

− recommended storage temperature;

− the ABO blood group;

123

- volume of content and average number of platelets;

- method of preparation including nature of additive used;

- donor/patient identity for autologous use;

- that the component must be administered through a 170 μm filter.

Storage and stability

1. *Platelets in the frozen state* should be constantly maintained at:

- -80 °C if stored in an electrical freezer;

- -150 °C if stored in vapour phase liquid nitrogen.

If storage must be extended for more than one year, storage at -150 °C is preferred.

2. *Thawed platelets* should be used immediately after thawing.

If short intermediate storage is required, the product should be stored at 22 °C ± 2 °C with adequate agitation.

Quality assurance

Demonstration of the swirling phenomenon, based on light scattering by platelets of normal morphology in movement, may be carried out either as a separate quality control procedure or as a routine part of the issue and transfusion of these products.

As indicated in Table 13(a) with the following additions:

Table 17

Parameter to be checked	Quality requirement	Frequency of control	Control executed by
Volume	50 to 200 mL	all units	processing lab
Platelet count	> 40% of the pre-freeze platelet content	all units	quality lab
Residual leucocytes	$< 0.2 \times 10^6$ per 60×10^9 platelets	all units	quality lab

Transport

If transport in the frozen state is unavoidable, storage conditions should be maintained during transportation.

1.   Thawed platelets

Transport of thawed platelets is limited by the short storage time. Storage conditions should be maintained during transportation.

Indications for use

Cryopreserved platelets should be reserved for the provision of HLA and/or HPA compatible platelets where a compatible donor is not immediately available:

–   in alloimmune neonatal and antenatal thrombocytopenia;

–   in HLA alloimmunisation;

–   in bone-marrow transplantation.

Precautions in use

–   Suitable HLA and HPA compatibility testing should be performed when required.

-    Toxicity of reagents used in its processing and cryopreservation e.g. DMSO.

Side-effects

–   Non-haemolytic transfusion reactions may occur (mainly chills, fever and urticaria).

–   Alloimmunisation, especially to the HLA and HPA series of antigens, may occur, but the risk is minimal.

–   Viral transmission is possible despite careful donor selection and laboratory screening procedures.

–   Protozoal transmission may occur in rare instances.

–   Sepsis due to inadvertent bacterial contamination.

–   Post-transfusion purpura.

Chapter 18: Granulocytes: apheresis

Definition

A component consisting primarily of granulocytes suspended in plasma, obtained by single-donor apheresis.

Properties

The principal function of granulocytes is phagocytosis of bacteria.

Method of preparation

Leucapheresis by cell separator devices. Centrifugal flow methods, either intermittent or continuous, are used. Improved yields may be obtained by addition of a red cell sedimenting agent such as hydroxyethyl starch, low molecular weight dextran or modified fluid gelatin.

Labelling

The following should comply with the relevant national legislation and international agreements. The label on the container states:

–   the name of component;

–   the producer's name and address (clear text or code);

–   the presence and type of suspension and additive media;

–   the ABO group;

–   the volume of the suspension and the expected number of granulocytes;

–   the donation number;

–   the date and time of preparation;

–   the date and time of expiry;

–   that the component should be transfused immediately;

-    that the component must be administered through a 170 μm filter.

Storage and stability

This preparation is not suitable for storage and should be transfused as soon as possible after collection. If unavoidable, storage should be limited to 24 hours at 22 °C ± 2 °C.

Quality assurance

As indicated in Table 13(a) with the following additions:

Table 18

Parameter to be checked	Quality requirement	Frequency of control	Control executed by
HTLV-Abs (when required)	negative by screening test	all units	screening lab
Volume	< 500 mL	all units	processing lab
Granulocytes	> 10 × 10^9 per unit	all units	processing lab

Transport

The unit should be transported to the user in a suitable container at 22 °C ± 2 °C.

Indications for use

Can be used as an adjunct to antibiotic therapies in severely neutropenic patients and patients with chronic granulomatous disease.

Precautions in use

As there is significant red cell contamination, compatibility testing is recommended.

In immunodepressed patients, granulocytes should be exposed to an appropriate dose of ionising radiation before transfusion.

Side-effects

–   Non-haemolytic transfusion reactions may occur (namely fever, chills and urticaria).

–   Alloimmunisation to HLA and red cell antigens may occur.

–   Syphilis may be transmitted.

-    There is a significant risk of transmission of latent viruses (CMV, EBV, etc...) to an immunosuppressed patient.

–   Viral transmission (hepatitis, HIV, etc.) is possible despite careful donor selection and screening procedures.

- Protozoal transmission (e.g. malaria) may occur in rare instances.

- Sepsis due to inadvertent bacterial contamination.

- Post-transfusion purpura.

- Accumulation of hydroxyethyl starch in multiexposed patients.

- Transfusion related acute lung injury.

Chapter 19: Haematopoietic progenitor cells

Definition

Haematopoietic progenitor cells (HPC) are primitive pluripotent cells capable of self renewal as well as differentiation and maturation into all haematopoietic lineages. They are found in bone marrow [bone marrow cells (BMC)], in the mononuclear cells of circulating blood [peripheral blood stem cells (PBSC)] and in umbilical cord blood [umbilical stem cells (USC)] .

HPC preparations (from all three sources) are intended to provide a successful engraftment of haematopoietic stem cells leading to a restoration of all types of blood cells to a normal level and function in the recipient. The infused HPC can originate from the recipient or from another individual.

Properties

The size and specific gravity of HPC from different sources are similar to those of mononuclear cells (MNC) of whole blood. HPC are recognised by their colony-forming capacities in different *in vitro* cell culture assays and by their cell type specific membrane markers. The membrane marker CD34 was found to be a common tool for the successful isolation/purification of HPC and is routinely used as an indicator in the quality control of the preparations.

HPC are short lived in liquid *in vitro*; cryopreservation (below -120 °C) allows storage for prolonged periods of time.

The yield of mononuclear cells should be sufficient to facilitate successful engraftment in the recipient.

Methods of collection and preparation

All treatment of the donors required to obtain an effective HPC preparation should comply with the relevant medical ethical codes and be performed with informed consent of the donor. Performance of the tests for infectious disease markers should be done within the 30 days prior to the HPC collection.

A. Allogenic transplantation:
All requirements for donor selection and laboratory testing are applicable as for a normal whole blood and cytapheresis donor next to full HLA typing. If the donor can not meet these criteria, deviation is permissable only after the documented approval of the donor's and recipient's physician.

B. Autologous transplantation:

The requirements are in these cases at the discretion of the patient's physician. If there is any positive marker for transfusion-transmitted diseases all personnel involved in the testing, collection, processing and storage of HPC preparation should be informed prior to their involvement. Storage should ensure that there is no possibility of contamination of other components. All containers and material which have been in direct contact with the biomaterial involved in the HPC preparation should then be labelled as a biohazard or likewise disposed.

-     Bone marrow

Bone marrow is harvested by aspirating the cells from the cavities of hollow bones. Further purification consists of removal of bone fragments by filtration and isolation of the "buffycoat" cells after centrifugation. This technique, based on density, is performed without any sedimenting or density gradient reagents.

-     Peripheral blood stem cells

PBSC are collected as mononuclear cells by cytapheresis of a donor. The number of HPC recovered from peripheral blood is only sufficient for a successful engraftment when the donor is treated with growth factors prior to collection when the donor is treated prior to collection with agents such as growth factors.

-     Umbilical cord blood

Umbilical stem cells are extracted from fresh placenta via the arteries of the umbilical cord.

Additional purification/manipulation of components, if indicated, can include: removal of granulocytes and erythrocytes, reduction/elimination of malignant cells contamination in the autologous HPC preparations or of the number of T-lymphocytes in the allogenic HPC preparations to minimise Graft Versus Host disease.

Purging and *in vitro* expansion are techniques which are sometimes employed to obtain increased numbers of stem cells in the final component.

Cryopreservation and thawing

Cryopreservation is commonly a part of the preparation of HPC for autologous and for umbilical cord blood transplantation, caused by an interval between HPC collection and transfusion needed for the clinical treatment of the recipient.

The cells are suspended in a medium containing a cryoprotectant (DMSO) and protein (autologous plasma/albumin) and are frozen in cryobags in a programmable controlled-rate cell freezing unit and stored in the liquid nitrogen freezer.

The frozen HPC preparation is thawed by mixing in a 37 °C waterbath and transfused immediately. Washing, ultrafiltration of the thawed product or the use of other cryopreservatives can be future improvements in order to minimise DMSO toxicity.

Reference samples of HPC preparations should be cryopreserved and used for quality control. An inventory control system should allow the allocation and retrieval of any components and its reference samples.

Labelling

The label on the container shall have at least the following information:

-   the name of the component, bone marrow, peripheral blood progenitor cells, or umbilical cord blood unit;

-   the producer's name and address (text or code);

-   date of collection;

-   the approximate volume in the container;

-   the names and volumes of anticoagulants or other derivatives;

-   the donor identifier;

-   the intended recipient's name or identifier.

and before issue for infusion, to the previous data shall be added:

-   identification and date of processing procedures used when applicable;

-   storage temperature;

-   in cases of allogenic transplantation, ABO and Rh type of donor and results of unexpected antibody tests when positive;

-   in cases of autologous transplantation, the label should include "For autologous use only";

-   a biohazard label, if the donor has tested positive for any test of infectious disease markers.

Storage and stability

HPC are commonly stored frozen within a temperature range -80 °C to -196 °C as determined to be appropriate for the cryoprotectant used.

An inventory control system shall be able to locate any component or the quality control vials from that component.

Quality assurance

Table 19

Parameters to be checked	Quality requirements	Frequency of control	Control executed by
ABO Rh(D) allogenic	grouping	all donations	grouping lab
HLA allogenic	typing	all donations	HLA lab
HIV Abs	negative by approved screening test	all donations	screening lab
ALT (when required)	not elevated as specified by national authorities	all donations	screening lab
HBsAg	negative by approved screening test	all donations	screening lab
HBc-Ab (when required)	negative by approved screening test	all donations	screening lab
HCV-Ab	negative by approved screening test	all donations	screening lab
Syphilis (when required)	negative by approved screening test	all donations	screening lab
CMV-Ab (when required)	negative by approved screening test	all donations	screening lab
HTLV-Abs (when required)	negative by approved screening test	all donations	screening lab
nucleated cell number/kg bodyweight of recipient (BMC units only)	0.5×10^8 cells for autologous transplantation $> 2 \times 10^8$ cells for allogenic transplantation	all donations	haematology lab
leukocyte viability	>80 %	all donations	haematology lab
Sterility	sterile	all donations	screening lab

Time of engraftment is defined as the number of days taken to achieve counts in the peripheral blood of the patient of $> 0.5 \times 10^9$ granulocytes/l and $> 20 \times 10^9$ platelets/l.

Review of the cellular counts and leucocyte viability, together with a review of the engraftment times, will be a component of quality control for HPC collection, processing and cryopreservation of the facility.

For any of the procedures mentioned as part of the HPC processing a relevant and validated assay has to be performed.

Transport

During transport of cryopreserved HPC preparations the temperature should remain below -120 °C; therefore the units should be shock and spill proof surrounded with adsorbing material soaked in sufficient liquid nitrogen; the primary container should be wrapped into a leakproof secondary container not interfering with the cooling. The container should bear the labels reading "Do not X-ray", "Keep frozen", "Labile unique human transfusion material" and "Rush". The address of the transport recipient should be clearly readable on at least two sides of the package.

Indications for use

Aplasia of the haemopoietic tissue by disease or after high dose chemotherapy and/or radiotherapy.

Side effects

-   non haemolytic transfusion reactions (fever, chills, urticaria);

-   risk of viral or bacterial disease transmission;

-   toxicity of reagents used in its processing and cryopreservation e.g. DMSO, animal antigens;

-   graft versus host disease in allogenic transfusions;

-   sepsis due to inadvertent bacterial contamination;

-   haemolytic transfusion reaction;

-   HPC components shall not be irradiated and leukocyte-reduction filters should not be used during its administration.

Records

Records to be maintained include:

-   donor, family of donor and patient pre and post transplant;

-   processing, procedures and protocols;

-   compatibility tests;

-   quality tests;

-   storage and transport;

- infusion and possible adverse reactions;

- final disposition of the product, facilities involved and personnel.

Chapter 20: Autologous predeposit transfusion

Several autologous transfusion techniques may be useful in surgery. They avoid the risks of alloimmune complications of blood transfusion, and reduce the risk of transfusion-associated infectious complications.

Autologous blood components can be obtained from pre-operative autologous whole blood donations in the weeks preceding surgery. In selected conditions, red cell or platelet concentrates can be collected using a cell separator: the equivalent of 2 to 3 red cell concentrates, or 4 to 10 standard platelet concentrate can be collected in a single procedure.

Autologous blood components obtained from pre-operative donations should be collected, prepared and stored in the same conditions as homologous donations. For these reasons, predeposit donations should be done in or under the control of blood transfusion centres.

Acute normovolemic haemodilution is the collection of blood immediately before or even during surgery, with blood volume compensation, leading to a haematocrit below 0.32.

Red cell salvage during surgery is another means of autologous transfusion. Blood collected from operation site may be given back to the patient either after a simple filtration, or a washing procedure. These two techniques do not allow the storage of the collected blood. They are usually performed under the responsibility of anesthesiologists and/or surgeons.

This chapter deals with autologous predeposit donations, where autologous components are collected, prepared and stored under the responsibilities of blood transfusion centres, in close cooperation with anesthesiologists and surgeons, which is a necessary condition for their optimal development.

1. Selection of patients

1.1 Role of the physician in charge of the patient

In elective surgery situations where a blood transfusion is expected, the physician in charge of the patient, usually the anesthiologist or the surgeon, may prescribe pre-operative donations. The prescription should indicate:

- the type and number of components required;

- the date and location of the scheduled surgery.

The patient is informed of the respective risks and constraints of autologous and homologous transfusion, and that homologous transfusion may also have to be used if necessary.

1.2   Role of the physician in charge

The physician in charge of blood collection takes the final responsibility for ensuring that the patient's clinical condition allows preoperative blood donation.

The patient's status with regard to virological markers should be established before the final decision.

In case of contra-indication, the physician in charge of blood collection informs the patient and the physician in charge of the patient.

1.3   Informed consent

Patients should be informed:

- about the autologous transfusion procedure;

- about the biological tests, including virological markers, that will be performed;

- that homologous transfusion will be used in addition to autologous if needed;

- that unused units will be destroyed.

This information should lead to written informed consent being obtained.

In paediatrics, the information should be given to the child and the parents, and the parents should give a written informed consent.

1.4   Contra-indications of predeposit donations

Pre-deposit donation may be carried out safely in elderly patients. However, more careful consideration may need to be given in the case of a patient aged more than 70 years or with a life expectancy of less than 5 years.

Children under 10 kg should not be included in a predeposit donation programme. For children between 10 and 20 kg, the use of volume compensation solutions is usually needed.

Any active bacterial infection is an absolute contra-indication.

In patients with haemoglobin concentration between 100 and 110 g/l, predeposit donation may be discussed according to the number of scheduled donations and the etiology of the anemia. No predeposit donation should be done in patients with haemoglobin concentration below 100 g/l.

It is recommended that patients positive for the following virological markers should not be included in a predeposit donation programme HBsAg, HCV, HIV and (when performed) HTLV.

The presence of a cardiac disease is not an absolute contra-indication, and predeposit donation may be done, subject to the assessment of a cardiologist, if needed. However patients with certain unstable clinical conditions such as unstable angina, severe aortic stenosis, or uncontrolled hypertension should not normally be included in a predeposit donation programme.

1.5 Medications

Oral iron should be give to patients before the first donation and until surgery.

Any use of erythropoietin should comply with the product marketing authorisation.

2. Predeposit blood components preparation, storage and distribution

2.1 Blood typing and microbiological screening of autologous blood components

Blood typing and microbiological screening should be the same as the minimum required for homologous components.

2.2 Preparation of autologous blood components

The methods of preparation should be the same as for homologous components, but in a separate batch.

2.3 Labelling of autologous blood components

Autologous blood component labelling is specific. It is recommended that blood bags for autologous donations be different form those used for the collection of homologous blood. This can be achieved by the addition of a distinctive labelling system to the usual bags.

The labelling should comply with the relevant national legislation and international agreements. The label on the container states:

- the name and volume of the preparation;

- the producer's name and address (clear text or code);

- the composition and volume of the anticoagulant and/or additive solution;

- the temperature of storage;

- that the blood must not be used for transfusion if there is abnormal haemolysis or other deterioration;

- that the blood must be administered through a 170-200 μm filter;

- the donation number;

- the date of collection and expiry date;

-   the statement: "AUTOLOGOUS DONATION";

-   the statement: "STRICTLY RESERVED FOR:
    - NAME and first name of the patient
    - date of birth";

-   the statement: "COLLECTION NUMBER.......X" (chronological order);

-   the place and scheduled date of surgery.

In order to reduce the risk of misuse of the product, indication in eye readable form of the ABO and Rh(D) blood group of the patient in clear may be omitted provided it is shown in bar code form.

2.4   Storage of autologous blood components

Autologous blood components are stored under the same conditions as, but independent from, homologous components.

2.5   Distribution and transfusion of autologous blood components

Release procedures must include a confirmation of identity written on the components labels, on the prescription document and at the bedside.

Pretransfusion tests should be carried out as for homologous components.

Autologous plasma may be used as a volume expander until 72 hours after thawing, provided that it is stored in controlled conditions between +2 °C and +6 °C. Otherwise autologous components should be stored under the same conditions as their homologous counterparts but clearly separated from them.

Untransfused autologous blood components must not be used for homologous transfusion.

3.   Records

Blood transfusion centres and hospitals should both maintain the following records for every patient included in a predeposit autologous transfusion programme:

-   the date and type of surgery;

-   the name of the anesthesiologist and the surgeon;

-   the time of transfusion, specifying whether used during surgery or post-operative;

-   the actual use of the prepared pre-operative autologous blood components;

-   the concurrent use of peri-operative autologous transfusion techniques;

-   the technique and the volume of autologous blood reinjected;

-    the use of homologous blood components;

-    the occurrence of any undesirable reaction related to transfusion.

- the use of homologous block components,
- the occurrence of any undesirable reaction related to transition.

Part D: Laboratory procedures

Chapter 21: Blood group serology

General comments

The purpose of quality control in transfusion-related blood group serology is to ensure safety by providing a good and uniform quality and minimising errors. There must be a special emphasis on training of staff, assessment of staff capability, equipment maintenance and calibration. Monitoring storage conditions of test materials and reagents and documentation of all of these as well as repeat testing of confirmed positive reactions on a further sample taken to confirm the identity of the original positive donation. Errors may be classified in two major categories:

a.   errors of organisation due to incorrect identification of samples or mistakes in transcription or in filing of results;

b.   technical errors, due to poor quality of equipment, reagents or performance of the tests.

Quality control intended to avoid errors of organisation is achieved by checking periodically the respective procedures. A more rigid quality control can be applied to the technical procedures and corresponding recommendations are given in this chapter.

A general approach in quality control of donor or patient blood group serology is to compare ABO- and Rh-typing results with previous data. This will disclose errors of both categories. Classification of any error should be attempted in order to obtain more detailed information about its source.

Quality control of serological techniques should be based upon internal and external quality controls. The internal controls are ordinarily executed by the serology laboratory itself. Results of the controls must be recorded systematically and be regularly reviewed by the supervisor of the laboratory.

1.   Internal quality control

The quality control procedures in blood group serology are subdivided into controls for equipment, reagents and techniques. This classification is considered to provide clarity, in spite of partial overlapping, especially between controls for reagents and techniques.

1.1   Quality control of equipment

Equipment used in transfusion serology, in particular centrifuges, automatic cell washers, waterbaths, incubators, refrigerators and freezers should undergo regular quality controls (Chapter 23). Equipment for automated blood grouping should also be controlled systematically, according to the manufacturer's instructions.

1.2   Quality control of reagents

The quality control of reagents should detect deviation from the established minimal quality requirements (specifications). Such requirements have been issued by the Council of Europe for blood grouping antisera and antiglobulin sera. Summarised requirements are included in the tables of this chapter.

New minimum potency standards for anti-A, anti-B and IgM anti-D are currently being prepared. The potency will be equivalent to FDA standards.

It is assumed that an evaluation of quality is performed on samples before purchasing larger batches of commercial reagents. Prospective purchasers should expect potential suppliers to provide them with full validation data for all reagents under evaluation. The following control procedures serve as routine checking before use.

The quality control procedures recommended in this section may basically be applied to reagents used for manual and automated techniques. However, reagents for blood grouping machines may have special quality requirements and more detailed controls; these are usually supplied by the manufacturers of the equipment.

Table 21(a)   **Quality control of reagent blood cells**

Parameter to be checked	Quality requirements	Frequency of control	Control executed by
Appearance	no haemolysis or turbidity in the supernatant by visual inspection	each day	grouping lab
Reactivity and specificity	clearcut reactions with selected antisera against declared RBC antigens	each lot on first and last day of declared shelf life	grouping lab

Table 21(b)   **Quality control of ABO-antisera**

Parameter to be checked	Quality requirements	Frequency of control	Control executed by
Appearance	no haemolysis, precipitate, particles or gel-formation by visual inspection	each day	grouping lab
Reactivity and specificity	no immune haemolysis, rouleaux formation or prozone phenomenon. Clear-cut reactions with RBC bearing the corresponding antigen(s) no false reactions. (see also quality control of ABO- and Rh-typing)	each new lot	grouping lab
Potency	undiluted serum should give a 3 to 4 plus reaction in saline tube test using a 3% RBC suspension at room temperature. Titres should be of 128 for anti-A, anti-B and anti-AB with A_1 - and B cells; 64 with A_2 and A_2B cells	each new lot	grouping lab

Table 21(c) **Quality control of Rh-antisera**

Parameter to be checked	Quality requirements	Frequency of control	Control executed by
Appearance	as for ABO-antisera	as for ABO-antisera	grouping lab
Reactivity and specificity	as for ABO-antisera	as for ABO-antisera	grouping lab
Potency	undiluted serum to give a 3 to 4 plus reaction in the designated test for each serum and a titre of 16 for anti-D, anti-C, anti-E, anti c, anti e and anti-CDE using R_1r-, R_2r-, r'r- or r"r-RBC	each new lot	grouping lab

Table 21(d) **Quality control of antiglobulin serum (broad spectrum) used for the antiglobulin test**

Parameter to be checked	Quality requirements	Frequency of control	Control executed by
Appearance	no precipitate, particles or gel formation by visual inspection	each day	grouping lab
Reactivity and specificity	a. no haemolytic activity; no agglutination of unsensitised RBC of any ABO group after incubation, as in the cross match, with compatible serum.	each day	grouping lab
	b. agglutination of RBC sensitised with anti-D serum containing not more than 10 nanograms/mL antibody activity.	each day	grouping lab
	c. agglutination of RBC sensitised with a complement-binding allo-antibody (eg. anti-Jk^a) to a higher titre in the presence than in the absence of complement or agglutination of RBC coated with C3b and C3d.	each new lot	grouping lab

148

Table 21(e) **Quality control of bovine serum albumin (BSA)**

Parameter to be checked	Quality requirements	Frequency of control	Control executed by
Appearance	no precipitate, particles or gel-formation by visual inspection.	each day	grouping lab
Purity	> 98% albumin as determined by electrophoresis.	each new lot	grouping lab
Reactivity	no agglutination of unsensitised RBC; no haemolytic activity; no prozone or "tailing" phenomena.	each day	grouping lab

Table 21(f) **Quality control of proteases**

Parameter to be checked	Quality requirement	Frequency of control	Control executed by
Reactivity	no agglutination or haemolysis using inert AB-serum. agglutination of cells sensitised with a weak IgG anti-D.	each new lot	grouping lab
Potency	an IgG antibody, preferably anti-D, standardised to give a titre of about 64 to 128 by the protease technique, should show the same titre on repeated testing with different batches.	each new lot	grouping lab

Table 21(g) **Quality control of saline**

Parameter to be checked	Quality requirements	Frequency of control	Control executed by
Appearance	no turbidity or particles by visual inspection.	each day	grouping lab
NaCl content	0.154 mol/1 (= 9 g/1).	each new lot	grouping lab
pH	pH 6.0 - 8.0.	a. each new lot for buffered saline	grouping lab
		b. daily for non-buffered saline	grouping lab
Reactivity	no agglutination of unsensitised RBC; no haemolytic activity.	each new lot	grouping lab

<u>Table 21(h)</u> **Quality control of ABO- and Rh- typing**

	Minimal requirements for testing	**Control samples**	**Frequency of control**	**Control executed by**
ABO-typing	use of anti-A and anti-B (using duplicate reagents if reverse typing cannot be performed). These are to be regarded as absolute minimal requirements, made possible by the introduction of monoclonal reagents.	one blood sample of each of the following types: O,A_1, B	each test series or at least once a day provided the same reagents are used throughout	grouping lab
ABO-reverse-typing	use of A1 and B cells.			grouping lab
Rh (D) - typing	typing in duplicate using two anti-D sera from different batches; use of the indirect anti-globulin test for D^{u-} confirmation in donors, where required. If two monoclonal anti-D's are used, they should be from different clones, it must be ascertained that the system will recognise D variants.	one Rh (D)-pos, one Rh (D)-neg sample	each test series or at least once a day provided the same reagents are used throughout	grouping lab
Rh-phenotyping	typing in duplicate using two different antisera for each Rh factor.	for complete Rh-phenotyping: one sample of each of the following Rh-types: R_1r, R_2r, r'r, r"r rr and $R_1^{w}r$		grouping lab

Table 21(i) **Quality control of low ionic strength salt solutions (LISS)**

Parameter to be checked	Quality requirements	Frequency of control	Control executed by
Appearance	no turbidity or particles on visual inspection.	each day	grouping lab
pH	6.7 (range 6.5-7.0).	each new lot	grouping lab
Conductivity	3.7 ms/cm at 23 °C (range 3.44-3.75).	each new lot	grouping lab

1.3   Quality control of techniques

Provided that the quality of equipment and reagents fulfil the requirements, false results are due to the technique itself, either because of inadequacy of the method or – more often – because of "operational errors" as a consequence of inaccurate performance or incorrect interpretation.

The quality control procedures recommended in this section are focused on the techniques but they will of course also disclose poor quality of equipment and/or reagents.

Table 21(j)

Kind of testing	Minimal requirements for testing	Control samples	Frequency of control	Control executed by
a. Testing for immune anti-A and anti-B (in donors)	use of A_1 - and B-RBC	serum samples with an amount of immune anti-A and immune anti-B respectively above and below the accepted saline agglutination titre of anti-A and/or anti-B	each test series	grouping lab
b. Testing for irregular alloantibodies (in donors)	use of test by which clinically significant antibodies are detected	serum samples with known RBC-alloantibodies	occasional input by the supervisor of the laboratory and participation in external proficiency testing exercises	grouping lab
c. Testing for irregular alloantibodies (in patients)	use of at least – an enzyme test – the indirect antiglobulin test or manual or automated testing with equivalent sensitivity	as for b	as for b	grouping lab

continued...

Table 21(j) (continued)

Kind of testing	Minimal requirements for testing	Control samples	Frequency of control	Control executed by
d. Compatibility testing	use of at least - a saline test at room temperature - the indirect antiglobulin test or - manual or automated testing with equivalent sensitivity	as for b	as for b	grouping lab
e. Type and screen	typing – refer to Table 21(h) Screen – with a sensitive method such as antiglobulin test, against a panel of cells chosen to provide homozygosity for important antigens	as for b	each text series but at least daily	grouping lab

1.4 Quality control of antibody quantitation

For practical purposes, RBC antibody quantitation is confined to the quantitation of anti-D. It is recommended that this be carried out by automated techniques rather than by manual titration, the test serum being assigned an anti-D value expressed in international units per millilitre after comparison with a curve derived from standard sera. All sera should be tested in duplicate as a minimum, and all national and in-house standards calibrated against the international standard for anti-D. Records should be kept of the data derived from processing the standard sera, these figures should show no more variance than two standard deviations.

2. *External quality assurance*

The internal quality controls described above should be complemented by regular external quality assurance, i.e. participation in a proficiency testing programme.

In external quality assurance, proficiency tests, coded "normal" and "problem" blood samples are distributed from a national or regional reference laboratory to the participants, usually twice to four times a year. The exercise can be limited to compatibility testing, since ABO-grouping, Rh-typing and -phenotyping as well as alloantibody detection will be automatically included. The proficiency test panel may consist of four to six blood samples, the participants being asked to test each RBC against each serum (or plasma) for compatibility. The panel should be composed in such a way that compatible as well as incompatible combinations occur. The proficiency test may be completed by asking for titration of one or two of the detected antibodies.

In the reference centre the results are collated and accuracy scores determined. The results should be communicated to all participating laboratories (in coded or uncoded form, according to local agreement) in order to enable each laboratory to compare its own quality standard with that of a large number of other laboratories including the reference centre.

If no proficiency programme is available in a particular geographical area, the laboratory should arrange mutual proficiency testing with another laboratory. Although such an external quality control will not be as informative as participation in a comprehensive proficiency testing programme, it will be a valuable addition to the internal quality control procedure.

Chapter 22: Screening for infectious markers

1. General comments

The quality assurance of screening of donors for infectious markers is particularly important and implies both general and specific approaches. Only validated tests that have been licenced or authorised by the responsible Health Authorities may be used.

There must be special emphasis on training of staff, assessment of staff capability, maintenance and calibration of equipment, monitoring of storage conditions of test materials and reagents, with documentation of all these actions. It is useful to include in the screening test an additional weak positive serum to check the sensitivity of the system. Repeat testing of confirmed positive reactions on a further sample, taken to confirm the identity of the original positive donation, should be carried out.

The specific approach to quality of the screening must rely on four categories of measures.

a. Internal, day-to-day quality control covering both reagents and techniques.

b. External quality checks, in particular confirmation of positive findings as well as confirmation of negative results where this is thought to be necessary in the setting up of a new technique or the testing of new reagents. Such confirmation should be carried out by the appropriate microbiological reference laboratory.

c. Occasional internal exercises, using a panel of sera which have been built up by comparison with standards available.

d. External proficiency exercises, involving the testing of a panel of sera circulated to laboratories by an approved reference institution.

2. Quality control of HIV testing

All current tests suitable for donor screening are based on the detection of antibody to the current strains of HIV. Tests are conventionally supplied in kits, using microplates or beads with the inclusion of negative and positive controls in each plate or run. The minimum performance requirement is the correct determination of these controls. It is further recommended that the tests include an internal weak positive control made by each laboratory by diluting a known positive sample in order to check for the reproducibility of the borderline signals.

Initially reactive samples must be subjected to repeat testing by the same technique by the screening laboratory. A repeat reactive test is a test with at least two positive results out of three. If both repeat tests are negative, the blood and blood components connected to this donation may be released for issue and use. Samples which are repeat reactive should be sent to the appropriate reference laboratory for confirmation. A check on the identity of the index donation should be carried out by testing a sample taken from the unit of blood linked to the repeat reactive sample.

Ideally confirmatory tests should be as sensitive as and more specific than those used for screening. However, some screening tests are more sensitive than the available confirmation tests. The technique currently most likely to meet the above requirements is Western blot, the sensitivity and specificity of which may be improved by using standardised amounts of appropriate antigenic epitopes provided as synthetic peptides or recombinant proteins. Immunofluorescence tests are available as an alternative confirmatory test to the Western blot. Tests for HIV antigen and the use of the Polymerase Chain Reaction (PCR) technology may be of value in the interpretation of doubtful anti-HIV tests. The confirmatory test should be repeated on a fresh sample taken 4 weeks after the first.

Table 22(a)

Parameter to be checked	Quality requirement (specification)	Frequency of control	Control executed by
HIV-abs screening sensitivity	detection of weak pos. serum	each plate/run	screening lab

3.   Quality control of HBsAg Testing

All blood or blood components collected must be tested by an approved test which will detect at least 0.5mg/mL for Hepatitis B surface Antigen (HBsAg). The operating principles and requirements are similar to those indicated above for HIV screening. Confirmation of HBsAg reactivity must include specific neutralisation and may be supplemented by testing for anti-HBc and HBe antigen/antibody.

Table 22(b)

Parameter to be checked	Quality requirement (specification)	Frequency of control	Control executed by
HBsAg screening test	pos. with 1ng/mL standard	2 tests/run	screening lab

4. Quality control of HCV testing

The operating principles and requirements are similar to those indicated above for HIV screening.

The confirmation of positive screening results is currently performed by immunoblot using several recombinant HCV antigens and controls. PCR technology is of value in the interpretation of difficult cases.

Table 22(c)

Parameter to be checked	Quality requirement (specification)	Frequency of control	Control executed by
HCV-ab screening sensitivity	detection of weak pos. serum	each plate/run	screening lab

5. Quality control of syphilis testing

There is a continuing discussion over the need for a test for syphilis on blood donors, but the test may be used as an indicator of risk behaviours for sexually transmitted diseases and is still required by most countries. Most centres use either a cardiolipin test employing a lecithin-based antigen either manually or on blood grouping machines, or a test employing a variant of the Treponema pallidum haemagglutinin test (TPHA). An ELISA test is occasionally used. Positive syphilis screening results must ideally be confirmed by TPHA, fluorescent Treponema antibody test (FTA), or Treponema pallidum immobilisation test (TPI).

The relatively complex nature of syphilis serology means that a wide panel of sera from cases of different types must be used in occasional external quality control and in the assessment panel of sera must contain at least one sample from an early untreated case of syphilis, and one from a treated case. Each type of serum in the panel must be tested at differing dilutions, and the new reagent adjusted to afford the maximum chance of detecting a positive reaction.

Table 22(d)

Parameter to be checked	Quality requirement (specification)	Frequency of control	Control executed by
Lecithin-based reagent and TPHA reagents	detection of weak pos. serum	minimum – start and end of run	grouping lab or screening lab
New reagent batch	detection of panel of pos. sera	each batch	screening lab

6. Quality control of malarial antibody testing

The only test currently available which is suitable for routine use in a transfusion centre is the indirect fluorescent antibody technique (IFAT), employing slides coated with malarial antigen. Any testing requires integration with local approaches to donor history taking (see Chapter 1).

Table 22(e)

Parameter to be checked	Quality requirement (specification)	Frequency of control	Control executed by
Malarial IFAT test – each antigen	detection of weak pos. serum (titre 1/20)	each run	screening lab

7. Quality control of cytomegalovirus (CMV) testing

Testing for CMV antibody is most commonly performed using ELISA and Latex particle agglutination test. There are two reasons for testing for antibody to CMV.

a. The screening of all donations for CMV negativity, to enable the building up of a panel of CMV negative donations for use in highly susceptible patients.

b. The screening for donations with a high titre of CMV antibody which would be suitable for making therapeutic immunoglobulin.

Control of the screening procedure employed will obviously depend upon the desired end product, but is achieved by logical choice of titre in the positive control sample.

Table 22(f)

Parameter to be checked	Quality requirement (specification)	Frequency of control	Control executed by
CMV-ab screening test	neg. with control serum titre 1/30	each tray or run	screening lab
High titre CMV-ab donor screening test	pos. with control serum titre 1/128	each tray or run	screening lab

8. Quality control of HTLV testing

In any country where HTLV testing has been implemented the operating principles and requirements are similar to those indicated above for HIV screening.

The confirmation of positive screening results is currently performed by immunoblotting and PCR techniques.

Table 22(g)

Parameter to be checked	Quality requirement (specification)	Frequency of control	Control executed by
HTLV-abs screening sensitivity	detection of weak pos. serum	each plate/run	screening lab

9. Quality control of HBc Ab

In any country where HBc Ab testing has been implemented, the operating principles and requirements are similar to those indicated above for HIV screening, with the exception that no specific confirmatory test for HBc Ab is available.

Table 22(h)

Parameter to be checked	Quality of requirement (specification)	Frequency of control	Control executed by
HBc-antibody screening sensitivity	detection of weak pos. serum	each plate/run	screening lab

10.   Quality control of ALT testing

Where this is performed, estimations should be by a validated technique employing high and low standards on each run. It is recommended that interpretation of the test on donors be based on a locally established normal range.

Chapter 23: Control of equipment

A. Environmental control

1. Premises for donor sessions

When sessions are performed by mobile teams, a realistic attitude towards environmental standards is necessary. The premises should satisfy common sense requirements for the health and safety of both the mobile teams and the donors concerned, with due regard to relevant legislation or regulations. Points to check should include adequate heating, lighting and ventilation, general cleanliness, provision of a secure supply of water and electricity, adequate sanitation, compliance with fire regulations, satisfactory access for unloading and loading of equipment by the mobile team, adequate space to allow free access to the bleed and rest beds.

When the sessional venue is permanent and under the control of the transfusion centre, provision should additionally be made for proper cleaning by, for example, the use of non-slip, washable floor material installed without inaccessible corners, avoidance of internal window ledges, etc. Where possible, ventilation should be by an air-conditioning unit to avoid the need for open windows. Air changes, together with temperature and humidity control, should be adequate to cope with the maximum number of people likely to be in the room, and with the heat output from any equipment used. A temperature monitoring device should be installed and checked daily by the quality control division.

2. Routine laboratories

The same general principles apply as those suggested for permanent sessional venues. The aim must be to provide a comfortable working environment for the laboratory staff and this must also comply with health and safety regulations. Bench design, as well as flooring, should eliminate corners which would be difficult to clean. In addition to the control of temperature and humidity, excess noise must be avoided by the removal to a separate site of all excessively noisy pieces of equipment. Volatile and toxic materials must be handled in appropriate exhaust cabinets to avoid atmospheric pollution. A temperature monitoring device should be installed and checked daily by the quality control division.

3. Computers and electro-mechanical devices

These items of equipment may have special requirements such as a more precise atmospheric control or the provision of a non-standard or stabilised electrical supply. Such requirements should be checked with the manufacturer and secured before installation. Where special environmental control is necessary, temperature and humidity monitoring devices should be installed and checked daily by the quality control division.

4.   Blood processing laboratories

At transfusion centre level, blood component production may be either a closed process, as in the case of the separation of cells and plasma in a multiple bag system, or open, as in the case of washed red cells. A closed process may safely be carried out in the normal type of environment described for routine laboratories.

Open processes must be carried out under stricter environmental control either by the use of laminar flow cabinets or in the pressurised system of a suite of clean rooms provided with air passed into the inner cubicle through high efficiency particulate air filters.

B.   Equipment control

Assessment of the performance of blood transfusion equipment must conform to Good Manufacturing Practice (GMP) and is mandatory on three specific occasions:

i.   on installation of the machinery, which must be accompanied by full validation data by the manufacturer;

ii.   after any repairs or adjustments which may potentially alter the function of the equipment;

iii.   if ever a doubt arises that the machine is not functioning properly.

In addition to this, a schedule of routine and regular checking of machine function must be drawn up, the interval of testing for each particular machine depending on two main factors. These are the frequency of use of the piece of equipment, and its expected "life" in the laboratory. Calibration must be performed regularly according to an agreed schedule, by designated personnel, to include the checking of the equipment itself used for routine calibration purposes.

Assessment of the efficiency of blood transfusion equipment may be either direct or indirect. A direct assessment comes from the carrying out of pre-determined checks at regular time intervals, aimed at the control of the proper function of the piece of equipment. Indirect information may be obtained by other quality control measures such as the proficiency testing of personnel. Satisfactory performance in this sort of exercise is an indication of not only adequate function of the laboratory personnel, but of the equipment they use.

Inevitably, different schedules may be designed for different types of equipment in use. Each piece of equipment should have an individual record where the type of control, the date at which the control was carried out and the initials of the performer are recorded. Each person using the machine and the supervisor of the laboratory concerned should be informed in writing of the control schedules, and the head of the appropriate department should check regularly that the controls have been carried out and any remedial action taken.

In addition to the performance of a regular schedule of quality control, it must be remembered that regular maintenance of equipment forms an essential part of quality assurance. Many of the larger and more expensive items of laboratory equipment are subject to maintenance contracts with the manufacturer; these maintenance contracts should be very carefully worked out between the supplier and a legal representative of the user, and adhered to strictly thereafter. Where no maintenance contract exists for a piece of apparatus, collaboration between the scientific and technical staff of the transfusion centre and the relevant engineering staff should ensure that a proper schedule of planned preventive maintenance is drawn up for each piece of apparatus, in addition to the schedule of quality control measures which will be carried out by the scientific and technical staff. The meticulous recording of maintenance and repairs is just as important as the recording of the results of specific quality control tests for any piece of equipment.

C.   Reproducibility of results

A check of reproducibility is based on two principal concepts:

a.   the determination of accuracy of the equipment by the testing of a reference standard;

b.   the determination of the drift occurring during the routine day by testing of working standards at intervals.

Since examination of reproducibility usually implies that the test concerned is quantitative in nature, it follows that numerical values can be obtained for each type of control applied. Graphic plotting of the results of tests for accuracy and drift should be carried out so that a gradual deterioration in performance can be quickly identified and corrected.

Where a numerical value cannot be ascribed to the result of quality control tests, reproducibility can best be assessed by the inclusion in the schedule of testing of appropriate strong and weak positive controls at regular intervals.

Proper education of the personnel using blood transfusion laboratory equipment is essential. The staff must know not only how the control tests are to be done, but why they must be done, and they should be fully instructed not only in the performance of quality control tests but in the rapid detection of departures from the norm. In almost every case, normal functioning of the machine is defined by the manufacturer and confirmed at assessment on installation. Meticulous charting of quality control measures will be the best method of quick recognition of deterioration in function.

Table 23 lists some of the equipment used routinely in blood transfusion practice and the minimum requirements for their control. Other items of equipment, for example automated blood grouping machines, automated blood processing systems, etc. require the design of specific quality control procedures.

D.   Data processing systems

Electronic data processing systems are being used increasingly in blood centres for information management and storage and as tools for operational decision-making and control. Because these uses are critical to product and quality, these systems must be fully validated to ensure that they meet predetermined specifications for their functions, that they correctly preserve data integrity, and that their use is properly integrated into the centre's operating procedures. The developers of computer systems used in blood centres should follow established principles of software engineering design to develop, document and validate all source codes. Additional validation in the blood centre, at a minimum, should include provision of a written description of the system elements and their functions, and on-line performance testing of the system under limiting or boundary conditions. A record should be kept of the validation testing.

Table 23

Equipment	Method of control	Frequency of control	Control executed by
Blood bag refrigerator, cold room, Freezer containing transfusates	graphic recorder plus independent audible and visual alarm for appropriate high and low temperature parameters	daily	technician
Laboratory refrigerator, Laboratory freezer, incubators, water baths	thermometer, precision thermometer. "Semi-annually" refers to the precision thermometer	daily semi-annually	technician technician
Blood bag centrifuge	precision RPM meter plus stopwatch to control speed, acceleration and retardation	bi-monthly	engineering
Table centrifuge	RPM meter plus stopwatch to control speed, acceleration and retardation	occasionally	technician
Antiglobulin test automatic washer	anti-D sensitised cells	every run	technician
Haemoglobin photometer	calibration standard Hb quality control sample	daily monthly	technician technician technician
Cell counters	calibration: reference sample. drift: working standard	daily	technician technician

continued...

Table 23 (continued)

Equipment	Method of control	Frequency of control	Control executed by
Automatic pipettes	dye- or isotope-labelled protein (1% variation allowed)	each batch of tips	technician
Balance	analytical-control weights 5 mg - 100 g preparative control weights 100 mg - 100 g	semi-annually	technician
pH meter	control solutions pH 4-7, 7-10	each time of use	technician
Platelet agitator	thermometer frequency of agitation	daily monthly	technician technician
Laminar flow hood and sterile area filters	air pressure meter particle counter	daily tri-monthly	user micro-biologist
Blood mixer (swing)	control weighing and mixing	bi-monthly	engineering
Spring balance for bags	control weighing	monthly	engineering
Blood bag tube sealer and sterile connecting device	pressure on bag and tube	every bag	technician
Blood transport container	minimum/maximum thermometer or a temperature recording device	every time of use (on receipt)	technician

Chapter 24: Record keeping

With records of results of quality control procedures a distinction should be made between records of results which may require prompt or almost immediate correction, and records of results which can only be evaluated statistically or by summing up over a certain period.

Examples of the former are given throughout the preceding chapters. Most typical examples are those where a quality control procedure is prescribed for each unit of a blood product or for each laboratory procedure.

Examples of the latter records (summary records) are given below. The director of the transfusion service or a specially designated person should evaluate statistical variations from the usual pattern or from given normal values. Evaluation may take place monthly or quarterly, and annually.

Rejection or deferral of blood donors (numbers, reasons).

Donor reactions (numbers, sex, age, reaction category).

Unsatisfactory donations (numbers, category).

Positive tests for infectious markers (numbers, specific, false).

Discarded units of blood and blood components (numbers, categories, reasons).

Outdating of units of blood and blood components (for each category, the outdating as a percentage of the number of usable units).

Transfusion complications (numbers, category) including transfusion transmitted infection.

External complaints (number, origin, category).

Clerical errors (numbers, category).

There are a number of other records which are important in transfusion centres but which do not deal directly with quality control. Examples are: routine working documents, blood group documents for patients and donors, the proportion of cross-matched units to used (transfused) units of blood products, statistics of issue and return of blood units, etc. Many of these records are mainly used for administrative or organisational purposes.

It is essential that the recording system ensures a continuity of documentation of all procedures performed, from the blood donor to the recipient, i.e. each significant step should be recorded in a manner that permits tracing in either direction of a product or procedure from the first step to final disposition.

Specific consideration must be given to the ability to determine rapidly;

- each patient's history of transfusion including the reason for transfusion and the record of all components;

- the identity of the donors;

- each donor's history of donation;

- the final disposition (including the identity of the recipient) of all components from every donation.

Records of quality control procedures must include identification of the person(s) performing the tests or procedures. Any corrective action taken must also be recorded. If corrections in records are necessary, the original recording must not be obliterated, but must remain legible. Records of quality control procedures should be signed by the supervisor.

Records should be kept for a period according to local or national requirements. It is considered that the retention period should be at least five years.

Retention of samples

Retention of donor samples for a period of time may provide useful information. The provision of such systems is contingent on the availability of adequate human and financial resources.

Part E: Transfusion practices

Chapter 25: Pretransfusion measures

1. Identification of patient at blood sampling

Samples for blood typing and compatibility testing must have a clear-cut identification. The following rules are recommended.

The patient identification shall be indicated on the tube label before the sample is drawn. Family name and given name and birthdate will serve as a minimal requirement for identification. Normally it should be supplemented by a unique, new medical identification. In newborn infants, the sex and the number on the identification wrist band is noted in addition. In patients with unknown identity, a unique series of numbers may be used on wrist bands and attached to the patient according to specified rules.

In immediate relation to sampling, the data on the tube label must be checked either by asking the patient to tell his/her name and birthdate, or by reading these or other data on a wrist band securely attached to the patient. This identity control shall be done even if the patient is known to the phlebotomist, who with his/her signature on the order form shall certify that it has been performed.

2. Blood group serological investigations

These include blood typing, antibody screening and compatibility testing before transfusion of red cell products.

i. Blood typing

The ABO and Rh(D) blood type and, when needed, other blood types, shall be performed before transfusions except in emergencies when a delay may be life-threatening and typing may be carried out in parallel with transfusion of the blood components. It is further recommended that antibody screening for the detection of irregular erythrocyte antibodies be carried out in conjunction with patient blood typing.

The normal procedure shall be to make the investigation in due time before expected transfusions, e.g. in elective surgery.

The laboratory must have a reliable and validated procedure for blood typing which will include double-checking of data at the time of issuing a report on the blood group, and other serological findings, for inclusion in the patient's clinical record.

ii. Compatibility testing

The compatibility between donor and recipient must be assured in transfusions of components containing amounts of red cells visible to the naked eye.

Ideally compatibility testing should be carried out on repeat samples other than the one used in initial blood typing but should, in any case, be carried out on a sample taken no more than 4 days before the proposed transfusion.

The basis for compatibility is a correctly determined ABO and RH (D) blood type in donor and recipient. When irregular erythrocyte antibodies are present in the patient's circulation, only red cells which lack the corresponding antigens should be selected for transfusion.

Compatibility testing between donor red cells and recipient's serum shall be done in all cases with irregular erythrocyte antibodies. It is recommended as a routine procedure even when no antibodies have been found but may be omitted if other measures (e.g. type and screen, see below) are taken to guarantee safety. The compatibility testing shall include a sufficiently reliable and validated technique to guarantee detection of irregular erythrocyte antibodies, such as the indirect antiglobulin technique.

A type and screen procedure, where used as a replacement for compatibility testing, must include:

1.   a reliable and validated, preferably by computer, checking procedure when the blood units are delivered;

2.   test cells which cover all antigens, preferably homozygous, corresponding to the vast majority of clinically important antibodies;

3.   sufficiently sensitive techniques for the detection of erythrocyte antibodies;

4.   Laboratory records of tests performed and of the disposition of all units handled (including patient identification).

Chapter 26: Transfusion

1. Safety measures

The medical person who gives the transfusion to a patient is responsible for the control of identity and other safety measures.

Verification of identity shall be carried out either by asking the patient to tell his/her name and birthdate or by reading these or other identification details on a wrist-band which has been attached to the patient according to well-specified rules.

Verification that the relevant infusion operators are being used according to manufacturer's recommendations shall be carried out by a medical officer before attaching the blood components unit. It is recommended that no transfusion sets be used for more than 6 hours.

Verification of compatibility between patient and blood unit shall be carried out by:

1. comparing the identity information received from the patient with data on the laboratory's certificate of compatibility testing (if appropriate);

2. checking the certificate of the patient's blood group against the blood group denoted on the blood unit label; and

3. checking that the expiry date of the blood unit has not been passed.

The identification number and nature of the units transfused shall be noted in the patient's record so that the donors can be traced if necessary.

2. Clinical surveillance

During transfusion of blood components careful observation of the patient is mandatory. This applies particularly in the early stages of the transfusion where significant transfusion reactions are more likely to occur and in the transfusion of any component prepared by an open system.

Blood components should be transfused within the recommended time to avoid compromising clinical effectiveness, safety and ease of administration.

3. Warming of blood

Rapid transfusion of cold blood may in itself be dangerous. Any warming device used must be controlled and monitored to ensure that the correct temperature of the blood has been achieved.

4. Addition of drugs or infusion solution to blood

Because of the risk of damage to the blood constituents no drugs or infusion solutions may be added to blood units unless it has been clearly shown that the addition is not dangerous either to the blood or to the integrity of the system. In particular any solution containing calcium or concentrated glucose should not be added either to the bag or the infusion system.

5. Handling of frozen units

Frozen units have to be handled with great care since the containers may be brittle and may easily crack at low temperatures.

After thawing of frozen plasma the content shall be inspected to ensure that all cryoprecipitate has been dissolved and that the container is not damaged. Containers which leak must be discarded. Thawed preparations should be transfused as soon as possible.

6. The risk of air embolism

During blood transfusion, air embolism is possible under some circumstances if the operator is not sufficiently careful and skilful.

7. Transfusion complications

Transfusion complications include reactions and failure of expected therapeutic response.

As each transfusion of blood components is a separate biological process, careful notation and reporting of any observed reaction is the responsibility of the attending physician (see paragraph on "side-effects" under each specific chapter).

It is important also to determine the efficacy of the transfusion of the specific component by recording appropriate pre- and post-transfusion parameters.

Complications may occur either in direct relation to the transfusion or with a delay of hours or days. All serious complications shall be investigated, mild reactions according to the judgment of the responsible physician.

When a serious complication after transfusion of red cell preparations has occurred and the patient shows chills, fever, breathing difficulties, shock, or hypotension, back pain (which cannot be related to the patient's underlying disease) the following shall be investigated.

a.   Check that the ABO and Rh blood group of the blood unit label is compatible with the patient's blood group certificate. If irregular antibodies outside the ABO and RH systems are present, check if blood of compatible blood type has been used.

b. A blood sample taken before the transfusion (may be available at the compatibility testing laboratory), a blood sample taken after the transfusion, the blood unit with the transfusion set maintained in site, and the pilot tube shall be sent for investigation. It is recommended that this include a direct smear and a bacterial culture test of the content of the blood unit, a serological investigation for blood group incompatibility, and inspection of the blood unit for any damage.

In the case of repeated, febrile non-haemolytic transfusion reactions, the use of leucocyte-poor blood for subsequent transfusions is recommended, preferably after investigation for the presence of antibodies to leucocyte antigens. If it happens for prevention of febrile non-haemolytic reaction associated with platelets transfusion, non steroid anti-inflammatory drugs should be used.

Long-term complications may occur. These include mainly alloimmunisation and disease transmission. As this text is not intended to be comprehensive in this area readers are advised to consult appropriate publications.

There should be cooperation between the physician and the blood banks to facilitate investigations of possible transfusion transmitted infections and to provide medical follow up of recipient in cases where a donor is subsequently found to have seroconverted.

Appropriate follow up and patient counselling is also necessary when significant alloimmunisation against transfused cells may have taken place.

8. Hospital transfusion committees

A hospital blood transfusion committee should include representatives of the blood transfusion centre and the main clinical units with a significant transfusion activity. It is recommended that physicians, nurses and administrative personnel be represented.

The main goals of a hospital blood transfusion committee are:

-    to define blood transfusion policies adapted to the local clinical activities;

-    to conduct regular evaluation of blood transfusion practices;

-    to analyse any undesirable events due to blood transfusion and;

-    to take any corrective measures if necessary.

Establishment of hospital transfusion committees is to be encouraged.

Similarly, systems of audit of the clinical use of components will further enhance the efficacy of transfusion practice.

Sales agents for publications of the Council of Europe
Agents de vente des publications du Conseil de l'Europe

AUSTRALIA/AUSTRALIE
Hunter publications, 58A, Gipps Street
AUS-3066 COLLINGWOOD, Victoria
Fax: (61) 34 19 71 54

AUSTRIA/AUTRICHE
Gerold und Co., Graben 31
A-1011 WIEN 1
Fax: (43) 1512 47 31 29

BELGIUM/BELGIQUE
La Librairie européenne SA
50, avenue A. Jonnart
B-1200 BRUXELLES 20
Fax: (32) 27 35 08 60

Jean de Lannoy
202, avenue du Roi
B-1060 BRUXELLES
Fax: (32) 25 38 08 41

CANADA
Renouf Publishing Company Limited
5369 Chemin Canotek Road
CDN-OTTAWA, Ontario, K1J 9J3
Fax: (1) 613 745 76 60

DENMARK/DANEMARK
Munksgaard
PO Box 2148
DK-1016 KØBENHAVN K
Fax: (45) 33 12 93 87

FINLAND/FINLANDE
Akateeminen Kirjakauppa
Keskuskatu 1, PO Box 218
SF-00381 HELSINKI
Fax: (358) 01 21 44 50

GERMANY/ALLEMAGNE
UNO Verlag
Poppelsdorfer Allee 55
D-53115 BONN
Fax: (49) 228 21 74 92

GREECE/GRÈCE
Librairie Kauffmann
Mavrokordatou 9, GR-ATHINAI 106 78
Fax: (30) 13 23 03 20

HUNGARY/HONGRIE
Euro Info Service
Magyarorszag
Margitsziget (Európa Ház),
H-1138 BUDAPEST
Fax: (36) 1 111 62 16
E-mail: euroinfo@mail.matav.hu

IRELAND/IRLANDE
Government Stationery Office
4-5 Harcourt Road, IRL-DUBLIN 2
Fax: (353) 14 75 27 60

ISRAEL/ISRAËL
ROY International
17 Shimon Hatrssi St.
PO Box 13056
IL-61130 TEL AVIV
Fax: (972) 3 546 1423
E-mail: eurinfo@royil.netvision.net.il

ITALY/ITALIE
Libreria Commissionaria Sansoni
Via Duca di Calabria, 1/1
Casella Postale 552, I-50125 FIRENZE
Fax: (39) 55 64 12 57

MALTA/MALTE
L. Sapienza & Sons Ltd
26 Republic Street
PO Box 36
VALLETTA CMR 01
Fax: (356) 233 621

NETHERLANDS/PAYS-BAS
InOr-publikaties, PO Box 202
NL-7480 AE HAAKSBERGEN
Fax: (31) 542 72 92 96

NORWAY/NORVÈGE
Akademika, A/S Universitetsbokhandel
PO Box 84, Blindern
N-0314 OSLO
Fax: (47) 22 85 30 53

POLAND/POLOGNE
Głowna Księgarnia Naukowa im. B. Prusa
Krakowskie Przedmiescie 7
PL-00-068 WARSZAWA
Fax: (48) 22 26 64 49

PORTUGAL
Livraria Portugal
Rua do Carmo, 70
P-1200 LISBOA
Fax: (351) 13 47 02 64

SPAIN/ESPAGNE
Mundi-Prensa Libros SA
Castelló 37, E-28001 MADRID
Fax: (34) 15 75 39 98

Llibreria de la Generalitat
Rambla dels Estudis, 118
E-08002 BARCELONA
Fax: (34) 343 12 18 54

SWITZERLAND/SUISSE
Buchhandlung Heinimann & Co.
Kirchgasse 17, CH-8001 ZÜRICH
Fax: (41) 12 51 14 81

BERSY
Route du Manège 60, CP 4040
CH-1950 SION 4
Fax: (41) 27 203 73 32

UNITED KINGDOM/ROYAUME-UNI
HMSO, Agency Section
51 Nine Elms Lane
GB-LONDON SW8 5DR
Fax: (44) 171 873 82 00

UNITED STATES and CANADA/
ÉTATS-UNIS et CANADA
Manhattan Publishing Company
468 Albany Post Road
PO Box 850
CROTON-ON-HUDSON, NY 10520, USA
Fax: (1) 914 271 58 56

———————

STRASBOURG
Librairie Kléber
Palais de l'Europe
F-67075 STRASBOURG Cedex
Fax: (33) 03 88 52 91 21

Council of Europe Publishing/Editions du Conseil de l'Europe
Council of Europe/Conseil de l'Europe
F-67075 Strasbourg Cedex
Tel. (33) 03 88 41 25 81 – Fax (33) 03 88 41 27 80 – E-mail: sophie.lobey@seddoc.coe.fr